Halliday's DEEP LYMPHATIC THERAPY

Grace Halliday

F.L.C.S.P. (Phys), F.R.S.H., A.R.M.T. (Bachelor), S.A.M.T.A. (Life Member), A.N.T.A., A.N.T.A.B., A.S.O.R.T., DIP. S.M.S., C.T.M.

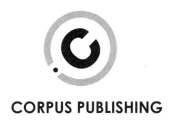

CORPUS PUBLISHING

First published in 2002 by
Corpus Publishing Limited
PO Box 8, Lydney, Gloucestershire, GL15 4YN.

Disclaimer
Whilst the information herein is supplied in good faith, no responsibility is taken by either the publisher or the author for any damage, injury or loss, however caused, which may arise from the use of the information provided.

British Library Cataloguing in Publication Data
A CIP record for this book is available from the British Library
ISBN 1 903333 08 3

Acknowledgements
I would like to thank the many people who have helped me to write this book, which I feel is the most difficult and time-consuming thing I have ever done. It is a lifetime of research, study and work after John and I had the 'incurable' rheumatoid arthritis and finding a treatment that it controlled and finally cured.

My thanks and appreciation of help, and for being there in my time of need to Wendy and Brian, Melissa, Rebecca, Kaye and Bill, John and Anne. Also to Stephen and Neela Walters who helped with the research, treatment, and that computer!

Thanks also to the many friends in England. Peggy Smith and Jenny Lidsey for giving me a home and driving me around in between consignments. Ann Hanks for doing extra computer work. Stan and Chris Duncombe, Valerie and Colin Smith, and Stephanie Syson for their interest and constructive help in many ways. Eddie and Marie Caldwell at the NIM College at Bury, and a special thanks to Eddie for the wonderful foreword to the book; Beryl Harper, our LCSP President, Lois Friedlander-Small and many others with whom I have had contact during my sojourn in England.

Also thanks to Lauraine and Alan Rainsforth and Simon Kneebone of Aldgate, South Australia for the work done with the computer and excellent illustrations.

Text and Cover Design Chris Fulcher
Drawings Alan Rainsforth, Michael Cheetham, Tim Fry and Simon Kneebone
Printed and bound in Great Britain by Bell & Bain Ltd., Glasgow

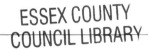

Dedication

This book is dedicated to the memory of my husband James Leonard (John) Halliday (1904–1965) whose love and devotion inspired me to continue the research and treatment, written to alleviate pain and cure other patients' complaints, as it did ours.

Contents

Foreword

The title of Grace Halliday's book belies its content. The book is not merely an account of Deep Lymphatic Therapy written (and re-written!) during the last two or three years. The study of and research into the effects of the function and malfunction of the Lymphatic System has been Grace Halliday's life for more than fifty years. This book is a distillation of a lifetime's work.

Grace is a self-confessed student and researcher, who has pursued her subject over the decades. An initial curiosity developed into an obsession and she has studied and researched her subject, including cadaver work, to enable herself to come to as thorough an understanding of the lymphatic system as possible. She has not yet achieved her goal and she is the first to acknowledge that there is still a long way to go and a lot more to learn about what she describes as a neglected area of medicine.

A therapist of unique talent, her patients are testimony to her skills. I have witnessed many of her treatments to patients with a wide variety of illness and disease. All have benefited from her treatments; some miraculously so. By treating the malfunctioning lymphatic system of these patients, Grace Halliday invariably brings about some improvement in them. Sometimes this improvement appears to be dramatic, even life-saving.

Grace Halliday is, despite a healthy degree of self-doubt, a remarkable teacher. She has been profoundly deaf for many years, but she is a marvellous communicator. She infects students and therapists alike with her enthusiasm and humour. She astonishes them by her knowledge of anatomy and physiology. She stimulates them by meeting every challenge and presenting them with her methods of examination and treatment for so many conditions. More than this, she also becomes their friend and mentor and carries on extended correspondence about patients and treatments with many therapists when she returns home to South Australia.

Perhaps the most valuable service that she has performed for the Northern Institute is that of allowing the students the opportunity to stand aside from traditionally accepted theory and practice and giving them the opportunity and the encouragement to look at and examine conditions and methods of treatment that are new to them.

At the age of eighty-three, Grace is still in a hurry to learn more. She is her own greatest critic and reviews and revises continuously and follows new paths of research with each passing month. She does not pretend to know everything there is to know about the lymphatic system, but what she does know about lymphatics cannot be matched by any other therapist. This book is Grace Halliday's life; it is also only the beginning of her work.

Eddie Caldwell, B.Ed. (Hons.), LCSP (Phys.), ACP
Principal of the Northern Institute of Massage

Instruction

A Note on the Use of Z instead of S

Corrections in spelling for the maintenance of the lymphatic apparatus

Fractionize	Neutralize	Liquefy
Fractionized	Neutralized	Liquefied
Fractionization	Neutralization	Liquefaction

The above is used to describe the action of the lymphatic system to break down any solids and bacterial debris within the interstitial fluid, propelled into the interstitium by the cardiac cycle – systole, diastole and diastasis cordis, through the fenestrated muscles of the veins and capillaries. The contaminants are fractionized, liquefied and neutralized to pure water before re-entering the bloodstream at the subclavian vein from the thoracic duct and lymphatic plexuses.

Lymphatic treatment is not distillation.

Neutralise	Fractionise	Fractionate	Fractionalise
Neutralisation	Fractionisation	Fractionation	Fractionalisation

The above spelling from dictionaries Oxford, Websters, Miller and Keane are used to describe the breaking down, or altering of a fluid and solids of chemicals, minerals by distillation. For example: vinegar from grape fluids, or apples to a cider and chemicals and barley proteins to produce whisky.

1. Lymphatic action on the foreign particulate or solid debris does not alter the interstitial fluid; it cleanses the original fluid for regeneration to pick up the proteins, minerals and carbohydrates in the bloodstream for redistribution.

2. **Distillation is altering the original fluid by changing it into something else.**

Introduction

This publication is written for 'hands-on' therapists to increase their knowledge and give relief to patients presenting with a variety of common ailments, often referred to as degenerative diseases, which have consistently been treated and cured during the course of my practice over the past fifty-four years.

Most of these problems are related to dysfunction of the lymphatic system which, if not addressed, consequently cause a malfunction and inability to remove wastes of metabolism, toxins and cellular debris, which build up in the various types of tissue. This results in a wide range of symptoms, presently named as diseases, all of which can be corrected by following the same basic treatment. A brief overview of the common factors observed during this treatment, particularly with my family, my husband and myself are as follows.

My first experience with arthritis was when Mother had the complaint in her legs and knees. She was about thirty-four years of age when she was immobilised. Both she and Father had a good basic training as vets from the early 1900s onwards. They didn't have any diplomas or certificates then but learned by practical experience from tending to their own farm animals and those of others in similar circumstances.

When she went to her Doctor, he gave her some 'medicine' which kept her very busy running between the house and the old Australian 'dunny' which was about four chains distant; this was to 'cleanse the system'. He then gave her some ointment with added menthol. The instructions were to rub the ointment into her legs and knees every day. Father, who had been accustomed to massaging horses' legs and knees for years, did the honours. After about three months of his treatment she recovered. The arthritic condition never returned to her lower limbs and she lived into her eighty-first year. The treatment was a bit rough but very effective. I kept that in mind.

My next observation was when Father killed and dressed two sheep for human consumption. When the meat was examined we found a chalky substance, much like a brittle bone, set in between every ligament in the carcase, from the bone up to the skin; we thought it had arisen from the bone. Because we were unaware of the origins of this condition, the meat was destroyed. These obstructions had created an uneven swelling and felt identical to the arthritic problems that had been treated earlier.

Fifty-four years ago my husband and I were destined to use wheelchairs for the rest of our lives. Our medical practitioners advised us to arrange for wheelchairs or crutches for mobility as nothing more could be done for us medically, to rest in bed until the pain subsided and take the prescribed drugs.

We had other ideas and began what I now see as a rough experimentation with massage and steam heat from wool blankets dipped in boiling water and wrung out. If one had the pain in a specific area, work was initiated at the origins of pain and relief was noted.

Steam heat was administered to the affected areas as above. We had to wring the foments out by hand in the early stages and used whatever type of glove made of rubber as insulation from the hot water. We used other types of materials, i.e. towelling or cotton materials but found they were not efficient because of burns and blisters. Wool blankets were the best and I still use them today when I treat patients.

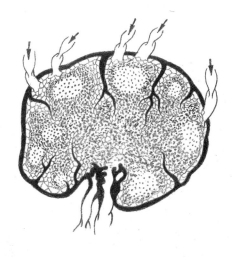

Figure 1: A typical lymph node.

From this humble beginning, the successful treatment of a then, to us, little-known system, the lymphatics of the body, was initiated, inhibiting the arthritis diagnosed by our medical practitioners and rendering the use of wheel chairs and drugs unnecessary.

We owned, and lived on, a property at Leawood Gardens, five and a half miles from Adelaide. On this property of a hundred acres, we grew chestnut, walnut and fruit trees; we engaged in floriculture as well as grazing sheep, cattle and horses. In addition, we operated a cartage contracting business carting crushed metal and sand from the local quarries.

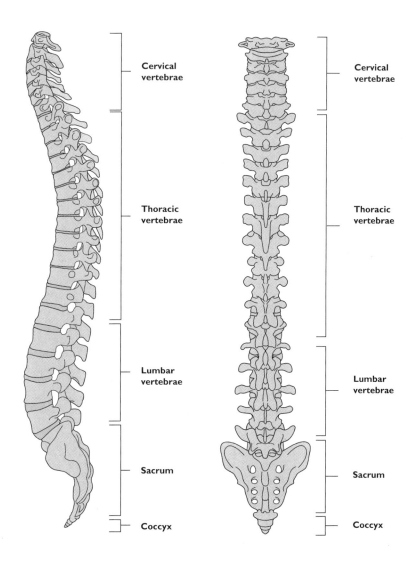

Figure 2: The spine showing the individual vertebrae; (a) lateral view, (b) posterior view.

Cervical vertebrae

Thoracic vertebrae

Lumbar vertebrae

Sacrum

Coccyx

Cervical vertebrae

Thoracic vertebrae

Lumbar vertebrae

Sacrum

Coccyx

Ten weeks after John was advised to get a wheelchair, he went back to driving one of the trucks. Similarly, I too, improved to the extent that I could work on the farm. When friends and relations observed our improvement, requests were made for treatment and they, too, had similar encouraging results.

We both had a working knowledge of home treatment. John's mother was the local nurse/midwife in the Stirling, Crafers, Aldgate and Piccadilly districts in the Adelaide Hills in the late 1890s and early 1900s. Likewise, my grandmother and aunts were nurses/midwives to Urania, Wauraltie, and Kilkerran on Yorke Peninsula, South Australia. Mother and Father, as previously mentioned, were vets. From an early age I was an interested onlooker and participant in the veterinary treatment.

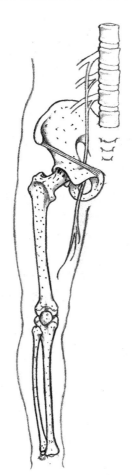

Figure 3: Haversian canals for interstitial fluid, blood, lymph vessels and nerve fibres. Volkmann's canals communicating with Haversian canals for the passage of blood vessels through bone and direction of drainage.

Before my marriage, I was a Police Officer in the South Australian Women Police. Part of my training included first aid, home nursing, judo and karate. Because of our work with a wide cross section of the community as well as training in observation of people, their physical characteristics and the way they moved, this training proved invaluable not only while in the Police Force but again in later years.

Through experimentation we found the greatest pain or discomfort originally appeared to emanate from the 'lumps' or 'runners' in all parts of the body. These obstructions appeared to be in between and down under the muscles close to the bone. Nerves, blood and lymph vessels lie along the periosteum before entering the small canals in the bone. When we worked, a stinging, burning, vibratory pain was felt until the 'runners' and 'lumps' finally degenerated with the use of hot foments and massage. In other parts, when pain was initiated at a site, it would traverse predominantly back to the spine. 'Bruises' were brought up to the skin, which were different to bruises from injury. The colour would be reddish brown at the onset, then about 24–36 hours later it would turn green, and at about the third day it would turn yellow, the three phases lasting about 5–5½ days before it faded. It appeared to arise from the bone. Blisters were also created from the steam heat, but they were not the same as an ordinary blister: the fluid consisted of water and an oily substance and would take about the same time as the bruise to heal. In tracing the pain, the 'runner' would be sore to touch, but at the end where the 'lump' was, the sensation was similar to an electric shock.

As we improved our technique, the discomfort from the work subsided and the problem, whatever it was, degenerated and disappeared permanently. Where we did not know, neither did we care, just as long as we had freedom from pain.

One phenomenon that followed treatment was vomiting. This happened to ourselves and friends alike. The vomitus consisted of brown sour-smelling strings and globules of slime, intermingled with greenish-yellow slimy waste, followed by a thick and colourless bubbly fluid; very little food, if any, was apparent. Approximately 1–2 pints (0.5–1 litre) of vomitus was eliminated. Variables influencing the quantity produced appeared to be the patient's size and the chronicity of the complaint.

Another phenomenon that followed treatment was an abnormal bowel action. The bowel wastes were black or brown, malodorous frothy 'sludge'. The vomiting on average would occur only once, maybe twice, with an acidic reaction of oesophagus and mouth. The bowel wastes elimination would occur up to 3–4 times in about three hours; the rectum and anus reacting to an acidic 'burn' after elimination. A burning sensation after urination was evident. The urine would be cloudy and had an offensive odour. At times it would have traces of blood in the fluid. The colour tended to be amber to a pale yellow cloudy fluid. If urine was retained in a container, a cream-coloured chalky crystalline substance would settle at the base and another slimy, darker layer above the crystal would at times have traces of blood in it. The third layer would be a cloudy

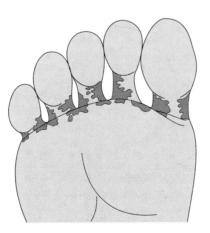

Figure 4: Blistering between the toes.

ammoniacal water. The elimination of this fluid would be immediately after treatment or up to three days thence. The blood in the urine was usually associated with the removal of the crystalline substance, which would lacerate the inner epithelial walls of the tubules.

An offensive body odour occurred after treatment, stale acidic perspiration, smelly feet, especially between the toes, and taste and smell would be similar to the detritus of decayed teeth in the mouth and nose.

With some patients, a blister would appear between the toes, the skin would turn white and lifeless. From 3–5 days later the blister would erupt, exuding a green-yellow pustular secretion. The top of the blister would lift off exposing the tissue underneath which would bleed. From the onset of the blisters to the healing stage, the patient would feel a burning, itching, painful sensation, which would last up to about six days. Depending on the chronicity of the complaint, the heels and soles of the feet would also be affected.

From my earliest studies it was difficult to differentiate between blood, bone, cellular, digestive or an inherited genetic weakness as a basic cause of the arthritic conditions in the body. Both homo sapiens and quadrupeds' rheumatic and/or arthritic conditions were identical. Bone and joint, hot and tender with uneven swelling, stiffness with a grating noise in the joints would occur as man and animal attempted to move. Loss of balance and mobility were also in evidence. Perhaps I was fortunate to have a good working knowledge of healing learned from my family.

In my early years on the farm, if an animal was injured in an accident or it had something organically wrong, my parents, with their knowledge as vets, would invariably cure the animal. Much was learned from autopsies if any animal died; as a result of these investigations many other animals were saved. When my husband had to seek help for his arthritic condition, we had no alternative but to use home treatment. He also had a good working knowledge acquired, or learned, from his mother.

After our recovery, I began studying, reading anything and everything that would possibly enlighten me as to why this ailment disappeared and allowed us once again to live a normal life. This study included taking notes from textbooks in libraries and the Adelaide University Library. This information convinced me that the substances, observed years ago while watching my parents attend to animals and performing autopsies, the deformities of bone, were identical to what was described in these publications. While treating humans and animals during the last few years my major observations of diagnosed arthritic problems were:

1. Humans had a basic mosaic pattern of hardened vein-like vessels with a high aggregation of hardened (or calcified) nodes, large and small, scattered between the vessels forming plexuses.
2. The lymphatic system is a network of vessels and organs to collect, engulf, liquefy and neutralize the ingested bacteria and foreign protein.
3. The blood capillaries and fenestrated muscles of veins distribute tissue fluid, also called interstitial fluid, into the interstitium with all the nutrients, minerals and chemicals necessary for the maintenance of bone and all cellular structures.
4. The lymph vessels, which are in close proximity to blood vessels and nerve fibres, pick up this fluid plus all foreign protein. The fluid on its way back to the bloodstream via the lymphatic and thoracic ducts is buffered through the lymph nodes and glands where the solid protein, dead cells, bacteria etc.are fractionized, liquefied and neutralized before entering the bloodstream.

In theory, we are supposed to have a bloodstream that is free of toxins and body wastes that contaminate the plasma and interstitial fluid being pulsated by the cardiac cycle through the fenestrae of veins and capillaries into the interstitial

Figure 5: Thoracic duct and blood vessels showing the direction of flow.

Figure 6: Deep lymphatic blind ending valved duct where the purified fluid flows back to the thoracic duct.

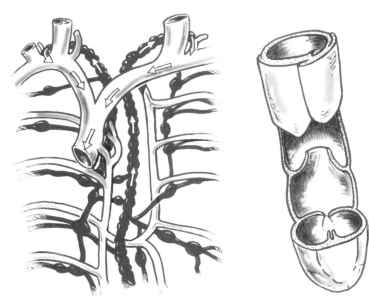

Figure 5   *Figure 6*

spaces. We should have a lymph system capable of fractionizing, liquefying and neutralizing the foreign particulate from cellular and bone cells. If the body has been injured pre-birth, at birth (as with forceps or mechanical intervention), in an accident or by any restrictions on tissues that will inhibit the flow of lymph or interstitial fluid before it enters the blind-ending valved ducts of the lymph system, the fluid gels to form an impenetrable barrier.

Lymph fluid relies on the propulsion created by the cardiac cycle: systole, pulsated through the arteries, veins and capillaries; diastole, the cycle which allows the blood to return to the heart cavities, ventricles and atria; and diastasis cordis, the pause before systole to allow the heart chambers to fill before the systolic pressure again pulsates the blood, a liquid tissue, through the blood vessels. Blood pulsates through a normal body at the rate of approximately 72–80 beats a minute.

Interstitial fluid is propelled back through into the blind-ending lymph ducts at 6–10 times a minute. As the interstitial fluid conveys the cell debris, dead cells, toxins, bacteria and any other foreign protein, it needs 6–10 propulsions a minute to build up sufficient pressure to push the above debris through the valves located in the lymph duct walls and the one-way valves inside the ducts. This action could be described as somewhat similar to a vacuum inside the vessels, which are activated by the expansion/contraction of the blood vessels. Illustrations of the above action of these vessels are of importance to demonstrate the simplicity of the exchanges.

As can be observed in the following chapters, the poisons of foreign particulate, ingested or inhaled, will drain into a lymph node where, to my knowledge, are fifteen natural killer and filtration cells. An enlarged lymph node with the above-mentioned cells was observed in solution at the second level, anatomical section of the Adelaide Medical School.

The foreign particulate, if flowing through the 8–10 nodes, normally will fractionize, liquefy and neutralize. If the drainage of fluid is slowed down by blockage to below 20 ft/second, a colloidin forms, a jelly-like principle produced in colloid degeneration. This degenerative substance will eventually form a plaque. The abrasive substance thus formed settles in between bone joints and deep in the muscular tissues. I have observed this in both humans and animals. It is a cream-yellow in colour, in plaques, and breaks like a chalk. It forms between the joints where the bones discharge the dead bone cells and other debris through the epiphyseal ends. If the interstitial fluid flow is insufficient to 'wash' the wastes through into the lymph ducts, the dead bone cells remain in the joints and the fluid seeps out by the compression of body weight on the bones. The bone cells and debris remain to wear away the synovial cells and the cartilage down to the bone, which then fuses. The nerve pain is excruciating and painkillers are prescribed. As I have noted over the many years of practice, the above condition can be reversed with the use of the hot pads and specific massage of the lymph vessels. The treatment is identical to what I do to treat any other obstruction or growth. Heat is applied initially and work is done to the affected areas, but not on the obstructions. Massaging around the epicentre to liquefy the wastes at the outer edge allows the interstitial fluid to pulsate into the area and the liquefied debris to be propelled into the lymph ducts. The process is painful in the beginning because the debris is too thick in texture and the patient feels as though whatever is moving is too large, too hard to flow through a vessel or too small as it stretches beyond its capacity. This phenomenon usually only occurs once.

Foreign particulate, which is plural, contains, or is composed of separate particles that are antagonistic to the system.

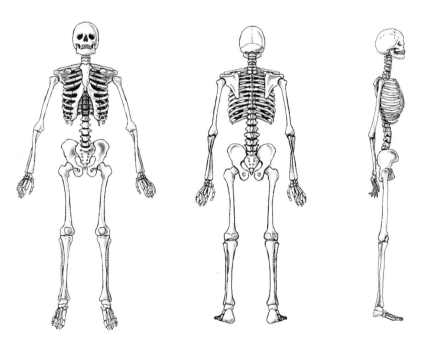

Figure 7: The skeletal system which protects muscles and organs.

Foreign protein is a protein deficiency causing weakness, poor resistance and swelling of body tissues (nutritional oedema) due to accumulation of fluid in the interstitium. I differentiate foreign particulate and foreign protein because:

1.   Foreign particulate is composed of separate particles that are not fractionized, liquefied and neutralized by the dysfunctioning lymphatic system; it is the precursor to suppurating and malignant growths, boils, carbuncles and other diseases (*see* osteomyelitis, page 121).

2.   Foreign protein, or protein deficiency, causes weakness and poor resistance to disease because of the accumulation of fluid in the interstitium. As the foreign particulate is not being fractionized, liquefied and neutralized by the lymphatic system, but kept at 98.4° in an airless environment, it will decompose. The fluid from the decomposed particulate is then distributed into the foreign protein causing growths, both benign and malignant and other life threatening diseases.

In 1991, while attending a conference in England, I saw a video made by Angus Strover, orthopaedic surgeon at the Droitwich Hospital, where he performed an operation on a knee joint to remove the meniscus. The fluid flow was copious in all directions, up, down and within the joint, which appeared to have opposing streams forming a 'whirlpool' movement to clear the debris. I work in the direction of the main flows, with the aid of the steam heat to liquefy the gel,

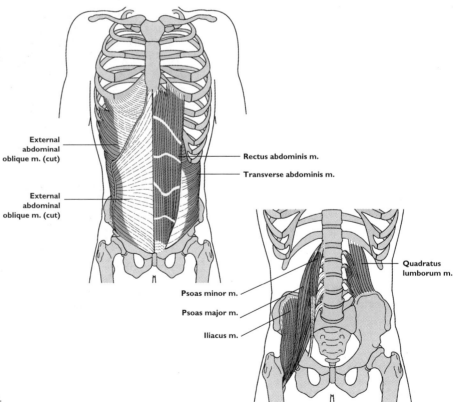

Figure 8: The obliquus muscles.

which helps to release the blockage in the plexuses. It is necessary to know in which direction to work. Although the lymph system is multidirectional, I find I get better results by following the main flow.

In lower back pain, treatment is not initiated at the spine where laminectomies are performed in the lumbar, sacral spines, but in the layers of obliquus muscles between the ribcage, iliac crest and the upper and lower leg.

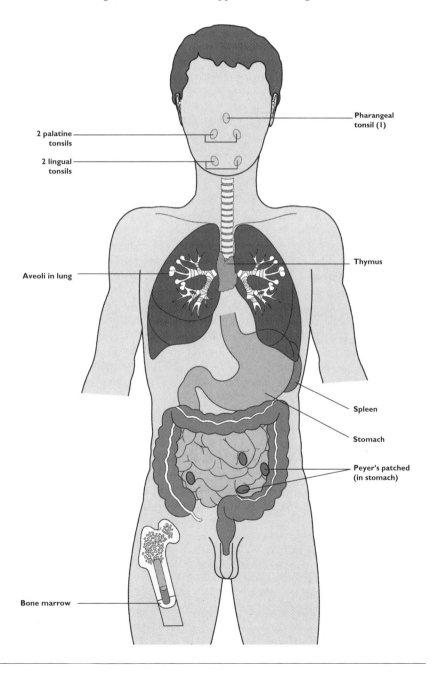

Figure 9: Some lymphoid organs of the body.

If the practitioner uses his/her hand held straight and curved at the carpal joint, and places the hand on the abdominal muscles starting at the lymph plexus under rectus abdominis near the umbilicus and pulls back towards the spine, several lymph plexuses can be noted which are joined together by small vessels or filters to form a barrier between the layers of muscle fibres that support the viscera in the abdominal cavity. Fibrillation of the nerve impulse from the brain to innervate the motor end plate occurs because the plaques of the blocked lymphatics are blocking the pathways of the nerves. The nerve impulse fails to complete the circuit between the ventral roots from the medulla to the motor end plate and the dorsal roots back to the brain. A stinging, burning, vibratory pain is noted in the affected area and felt mainly at the root entrance into the medulla in the spine and at the origins of insertions of muscles and ligaments on the femoral bone and ischium.

Part One

Origins of Lymphatics

Claudius Galen, born at Pergamon, Greece, 130–201AD.

The vessels are difficult to see unless injected with some visible material. In the living animal the vessels in the small intestines are 'injected' with fat after a fatty meal and appear white. Such vessels were observed in 300BC by Herophilus and Eristratus in the famous Alexandrian Medical School, but their function was not understood. Galen did not believe that these lacteals were different from arteries and veins and they were forgotten until the Renaissance, when a new spirit of scientific enquiry emerged. Gaspara Asselli, Professor of Anatomy and Surgery in Pavia, described in 1622 the appearance of lymphatic vessels in the mesentery of a well-fed dog. He traced the mesenteric glands and as a true disciple of Galen, he believed they went to the liver where the contents were 'concocted' into blood. In 1651 Jean Pecquet, a physician of Montpelier, described the thoracic duct through which the liquor of the 'milky veins' throws itself 'headlong into the whirlpool of the heart'. Soon after Pecquet's discovery, Rudbeck, Professor of Anatomy in Uppdala, described the vasa serosa in the liver. Bartholin, Professor of Anatomy in Copenhagen, found serous vessels in many parts of the body and in 1653 he called them lymphatics.

The number of lymph nodes amounts to an average of 60 in dogs, 190 in pigs, 300 in cattle, 8000 in horses and 450–500 in man. As regards the capillaries; it is neither the appearance of muscle fibres nor the two layers of the vessel walls of which the smallest lymphatics are still devoid, but the appearance of valves, which characterises them. As a rule, lymphatics cross on the way to the thoracic duct and the large vessels at least once, but frequently not less than 8–10 lymph nodes – lymphatics of the thyroid and oesophagus were observed to be drained by the thoracic duct. Great importance is attached to this fact in connection with the early metastases of malignant tumours. It is due to the presence of valves that lymph flow is multidirectional. Lymphatics are passable only in a centripetal direction. This rule is not always valid. If in pathological conditions lymphatics become grossly dilated by a **serious congestion** the valves become insufficient and flow is possible in both directions. This is why I stress that you must **not overwork**, through excessive pressure when doing massage. Only gentle flat hand massage must be used because the foreign particulate will block elsewhere.

Early Observations

In the general analysis and cross analysis of all the systems of the body that give life, general maintenance, reproduction, genetics carried on from the time of evolution, and generation to generation, involve much research into the interaction of cells of bone and tissue.

For many years we were unaware of the basic cause of the complaints that had been treated and why this particular method gave the desired relief. From my early studies it became obvious the system, which benefited most was that of the lymphatics.

When an obstruction in muscular tissue, or on bone in any part of the anatomy, the pain, swelling, heat, or whatever was emanating from the area, blood and lymph vessels, nerves, and muscles were traced. If this obstruction was not evident in a textbook, and on examination was causing discomfort, then it was a 'foreign body' in the anatomical structure.

In the initial stages of practice, my mind was clear of all the do's and don'ts of teaching that we must not touch nor treat, and if we did, drastic consequences

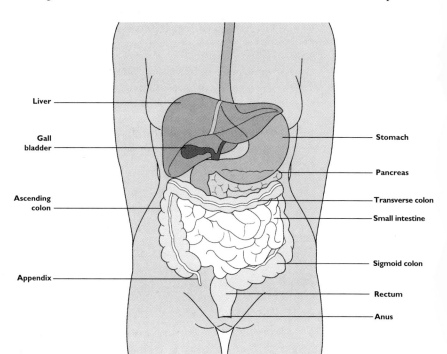

Figure 10: The intestinal organs with pancreas and liver. The villi in the intestines absorb the nutrition from the food ingested and deposits the lipids into the mesenteric vessels and portal vein.

would occur. Our logic was, if the 'thing' hurt, eliminate it by any means at our disposal. We soon learnt that if getting rid of the 'thing' was painful and left what we termed 'nerve pain', we had to re-assess our methods of treatment. Going through or over the 'foreign' body caused distress, but if we went around or under, the results were more favourable. By going around, it stopped the expansion of the tissues, and by going under, if possible, the small threads of roots would disintegrate; the 'foreign' body would be fractionized, liquefied and neutralized to pure water.

My first thoughts were:

1.   How did these obstructions form?
2.   From what processes of the body?
3.   Where and how did they originate?
4.   Was it diet or anything concerned with digestion?
5.   Our way of life and its subsequent knocks, overwork and overplay injuries, or any parts of the anatomy dysfunctioning, prevents other parts or systems from working efficiently.

Much information was gained from treating or experimenting on organs, muscles, ligaments, tendons and bone and noting progress; we also traced the pathways of nerves, blood vessels and lymphatics, noting their direction of flow. All my later experiments were conducted with reference to whatever textbook I was reading. If textbook and treatment complemented each other, the overall treatment improved.

I considered the digestive system to be of primary importance because so many problems could manifest from its dysfunction. Digestion begins in the mouth with release of acids, enzymes, and gastric juices activated by mastication from the salivary glands, parotid, submandibular, lingual and digestive glands in the cheeks. The glands beneath the tongue step up secretion and through the enzyme alpha amylase, they produce starches, breaking down some of the carbohydrates into smaller molecules known as maltose and glucose. The bolus of food is propelled down the oesophagus by peristalsis into the stomach, where the mixture of chemicals, mucus, hydrochloric acid and the enzyme pepsin is poured onto it. Alpha amylase stops working, but a new series of chemical reactions begins, triggered off by nerve impulses. The amount of stomach juices released is governed here and in the intestine by nerve impulses, the presence of food itself and the secretion of hormones etc.

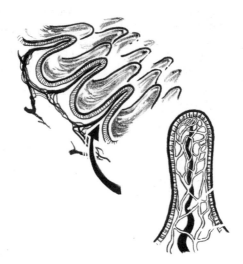

Figure 11: The villi pick up the whole of the nutrition from the bolus of food which is transported to the liver to be agitated to water.

The lipids are drawn from the bolus of food by the villi (*see* page 79) in the bowel and intestines, secreted in the mesenteric lymphatics, to be transported by the portal vein to the liver. Fats are emulsified by bile salts, bile pigments and alpha amylase and agitation. The emulsified fats are acted on by pancreatic and enteric lipase to form fatty acids, glycerol and mono glycerides which are absorbed through the intestinal walls.

If there is an imbalance of enzymes as described above and the lymph collection below, the application of steam heat would be important to assist in emulsifying the lipids. Lymph formed in the liver drains mainly into two groups of collecting vessels. A descending group accompanies the branches of the portal vein hepatic artery and biliary passages which emerges at the hilus and enters the hepatic nodes in this region. There is also an ascending group which forms around the branches of the hepatic veins and drains into the intrathoracic nodes around the terminal segment of the vena cava. In addition to these collecting ducts which drain the deeper lobules of the liver, there are also superficial vessels draining the peripheral lobule into the supraxiphoid nodes and nodes around the oesophagus and around the ceolic axis.

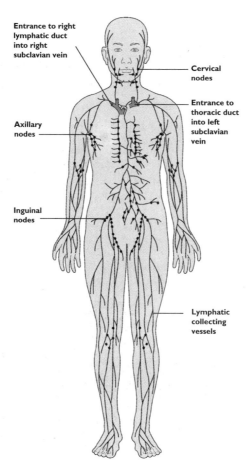

Entrance to right lymphatic duct into right subclavian vein

Cervical nodes

Entrance to thoracic duct into left subclavian vein

Axillary nodes

Inguinal nodes

Lymphatic collecting vessels

Figure 12: Indicating the overall lymphatic drainage. There are between 450 and 500 nodes in a body. Some of the more important ones are illustrated.

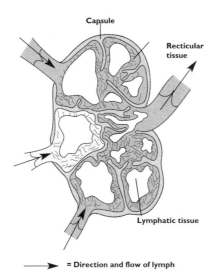

Capsule

Recticular tissue

Lymphatic tissue

⟶ = Direction and flow of lymph

Figure 13: A lymph node cut transversely showing the afferent and efferent drainage.

Lymph fluid must pass through 8–10 lymph nodes for the phagocytic action of the lymph cells to purify the 'foreign' matter and alien poisons discharged into the tissue fluid by tissue and bone cells during repair and division before entering the bloodstream.

If there is an imbalance of fluid and emulsified fats, patients suffer some form of discomfort and pain from indigestion, gastric upsets, deep pain in the region of diaphragm over the liver and under the pericardium. In the diaphragm there is a two-way flow of lymph:

1. Back through the crural muscle to the thoracic duct.
2. Over the liver and under pericardium to drain into the intercostals and axilla tails to the deep lymphatics axilla, brachial, intermediate and subclavian, and the lymphocentres of the supraclavicular fossa. Lymph also drains into the parasternal junctions.

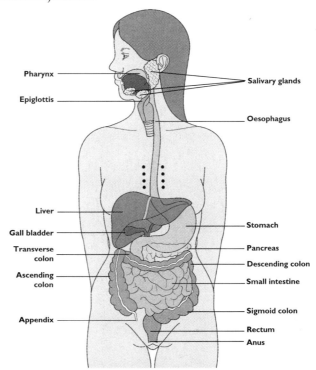

Pharynx

Epiglottis

Salivary glands

Oesophagus

Liver

Gall bladder

Transverse colon

Ascending colon

Appendix

Stomach

Pancreas

Descending colon

Small intestine

Sigmoid colon

Rectum

Anus

Figure 14: The digestive system from mastication to excretion.

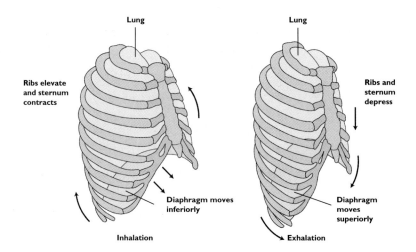

Figure 15: The respiratory system, inspiration, expiration. The epiglottis is the lidlike cartilaginous structure over hanging the entrance to the larynx. The action of glutition closes the opening to the trachea by placing the larynx against the epiglottis preventing food and fluids from entering the larynx and trachea.

Figure 16: The movement of the diaphragm on to the lungs at inspiration, expiration.

The deep lymphatics as described is a system responsible for the vagus nerve impulse fibrillation with a resultant angina and other heart dysfunctions, also lungs affected by inhibition of respiration/expiration caused by the fibrillation of the phrenic nerve.

If I suspect cholesterol accumulation, or if a patient has had a positive test for cholesterol, I work on the diaphragm, liver, pancreas, and bowel to release the oedematous formations. Then I work on the cheeks, and digastric belly to release the enzymes required to break down the lipids. My first observation of this condition was in the pathology and anatomy section at the medical school.

1. In pathology; an oedematous leg partially dissected by the students, a high aggregation of fatty obstructions on bone, in muscles and ligaments up to the dermis.

2. In anatomy; a segment of heart/aorta slice in solution – identical fatty obstructions lining the walls of aorta and heart.

Work has to be done in the direction of the lymph flow in liver and diaphragm, with the application of steam heat and the relief from pain is soon noted. After treatment, cholesterol tests on patients concerned by their medical practitioner show a decrease in concentration.

The lymphatics of bone structure would be of equal importance to digestion. This system is responsible for the many dysfunctions/malfunctions encountered by the complementary medicine practitioner.

The substance of bone is about half water and half solids. The composition of the solid matter includes white fibrous tissue for elasticity, calcium phosphate, calcium carbonate, calcium fluoride, magnesium phosphate and sodium chloride. Calcium in tissue fluid unites with free phosphate liberated locally in high concentration to form insoluble calcium phosphate crystals. Calcium oxalate gives rise to oxalosis and renal failure.

Anatomy of a Bone

Epiphysis = the end of a long bone usually wider than the shaft.

Metaphysis = the wider part at the end of a long bone adjacent to the epiphyseal disk.

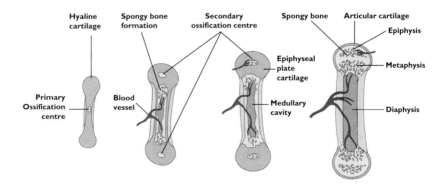

Figure 17: Anatomy of bone at different stages of growth.

Diaphysis = the portion of a long bone between the ends or extremities which are usually articular and wider than the shaft. It consists of a tube of compact bone, enclosing the medullary cavity:

1.   called also shaft;
2.   the portion of a bone formed from a primary centre of ossification.

Nerves, blood and lymph vessels lie along the periosteum before entering small canals in the bone. Calcification of arteries and arterioles are frequently demonstrable in X-rays. Vascular calcifications are usually not limited to where bone changes take place, but frequently occur in distant regions.

The large arteries are supplied with blood vessels, nerves and lymphatic vessels within the tunica adventitia, tunica media and tunica intima. If the feeding vessel to capillary/capillaries is interrupted, this extremely tenuous blood supply to the end point (bone cells) will be lost, which would result in death of bone no longer supplied by the blood. This has been observed when treating arthritis and osteoporosis.

The primary phenomenon is an osteolytic process which may be in the form of a large wedge taking up increasingly large amounts of bone substances, so that in a tibia, it extends to encompass the entire shaft in its transverse diameter. We see this wedge advance from above downwards until the whole longitudinal length of the shaft becomes involved. In the femur, a wedge advances from below upwards, following this wedge is an extensive osteoblastic reaction leading to a dense heavily trebaculated bone of irregular pattern. I have noted over the years of practice that periostal proliferation will be present and much increased.

A specimen observed in anatomy was a lower section of femur, the knee joint and a small section of tibia and fibula, cut in halves and in solution, of a woman who had died at the age of fifty-four years. This specimen showed the knee joint to be completely filled and locked by a substance. This substance had locked the knee a couple of years previously and had been released by surgery and manipulation under anaesthetic. The operation was not a success as the knee locked again after a few months.

All patients examined who suffer from diagnosed arthritis, multiple sclerosis and other associated complaints have an identical pattern of bone disorders and lymph drainage obstructions.

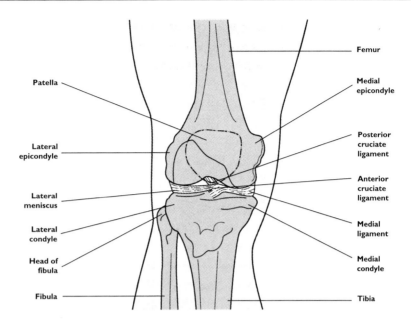

Figure 18: The knee showing placement of ligaments and bone.

A man in his mid-thirties whose foot I examined when he brought his son for treatment had an operation to remove a growth/obstruction from between the cuneiform and tarsal bones. After the operation he brought the specimen with him, which had been placed in solution. The chalky substance removed by surgery would have been approximately 2.5cms in diameter, and at the centre 75mms thick. The colour, pale and creamy, was the same as cloudy urine. It had no stability and had already broken into three pieces. I kept it for a month for observation, and at the end of that time it had disintegrated into many pieces and the residue held in solution.

A periostophyte is a bony outgrowth on the periosteum, which I observed many years ago on the skeletal fetlock of a bullock. It forms a 'splint' on the canon bone of horses and cattle.

The same outgrowth forms on homo sapiens periosteum and is called a 'spur'. The 'splint' on animals and the 'spur' on homo sapiens, with patience, specialized massage and steam heated pads, will slowly fractionize and liquefy the obstructions because it is a brittle bone structure with no stability.

An osteophyte / osteophyma is a bony excrescence or outgrowth, which is formed at the attachment of muscle fibres into bone canals. I observe this at the muscle attachments to bone where stress and strain will rupture or tear the tissue cells from the canals. The calcium in the interstial fluid enters the ruptured cells, and combines with the phosphate bonds released from the mitochondria of the tissue cells, plus the leakage of bone protein to form the 'bony excrescence'. Pain is exacerbated with treatment because of the fibrillated nerve fibres and feels like an electric shock. The condition responds to massage and steam heat.

The Dysfunctional Lymphatic System

Theoretically, we have a bloodstream free from toxins, debris or any foreign particulate, including drugs, which would be detrimental to the health of bone and cellular tissue. Also, a lymphatic system capable of fractionizing, liquefying, neutralizing and draining the wastes created by anabolism, metabolism, catabolism or any foreign particulate or protein either ingested or inhaled. If a body of homo sapiens or quadrupeds has been injured pre-birth, at birth (e.g. by the use of forceps) accidents or restrictions on bone or cellular tissue, a calcification manifests on bone and extends through the musculature to prevent free movement.

When the lymph nodes block from the above debris and the drainage is not viable, it prevents the natural killer cells and the agranular cells from fractionizing, liquefying, neutralizing the foreign particulate accumulated in the tissues or vessels before the purified water can be drained back into the bloodstream. To my knowledge there are fifteen natural killers (NK cells and agranular filtration cells) in the body of a lymph node through which the foreign particulate drains by propulsion from the pulsation of the cardiac cycle. It traverses through 8–10 lymph nodes to be purified back to water and plasma.

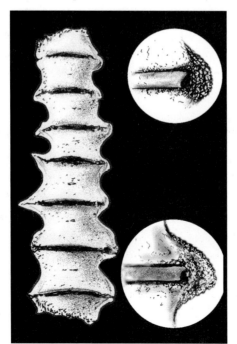

With the use of the steam-heated pads and massage in the direction of flow, the patient will be physically aware of the fluid pathways at the onset because the foreign particulate appears to be too solid to drain through the small vessels.

Figure 19:

With the liquefaction from the hot foments and the interstitial fluid flow created by the cardiac cycle into the interstitium, the foreign particulate will drain through the fine meshwork of lymphatic vessels and the multidirectional nodes and vessels where it is fractionized, liquefied and neutralized. The purified fluid will then drain into the blind ending valved ducts entering the thoracic duct emptying into the subclavian vein as pure water.

The three phases of the cardiac cycle are;

1.   Systole, which forces oxygenated blood from the heart into the arteries, veins and capillaries.
2.   Diastole, when the heart relaxes and allows the blood to flow back into the ventricles and atria.
3.   Diastasis cordis, the pause to allow all chambers of the heart to fill before the next systole.

Some patients only require one treatment for relief; others will need several treatments, according to the chronicity of the blocked drainage. Contrary to reports that deep lymphatic massage is harmful because it "increases the amount of fluid in the body", fluid cannot be increased because there is no ingestion of either fluids or nutrients while having treatment. There is only the feeling of extra fluid when the gelled and consolidated debris is liquefied from a solid mass to a fluid as it is drained away in the direction of flow. Water, when gelled or consolidated, will increase in volume and with the degenerative properties of the foreign particulate, will block any fluid draining vessels, fibrillate the nerve fibres in close proximity and constrict blood vessels through pressure to slow down the blood flow (stenosis).

Steam heat is essential for all deep lymphatic treatments.

Where there has been an accident with injury to cellular tissue causing bruises; rupturing of cells, blood and lymphatic vessels drainage and injury to bone, the interstitial fluid, which is half water, half plasma, will gel. The normal flow of twenty ft/second for the fluid has been slowed down or blocked by the accident. The calcium in the cellular tissue will seep into and mix with the phosphates stored in the mitochondria of the ruptured cells; calcification occurs and 'loose bodies' are formed. The 'white cloud or shadow' observed in X-rays and scans throughout the body and around the bones is the precursor to arthritis.

Most degenerative problems are related to dysfunction of the lymphatic system, which, if not treated, will cause the inability to remove wastes and other debris from the body. The above builds up in various types of tissue and causes a wide variety of complaints, which are called 'diseases', all of which can be treated and corrected by the same basic treatment.

The Deep Lymphatic System

The deep lymphatic system took over forty years of treatment and research to write. Some has been written in Part One, 'The Origins', 'Early Observations' and 'Dysfunctional Lymphatic System'.

To describe further the origins of the physiology and lymphatics of the anatomy, a start must be made at the ingestion of food and fluids required by the bodies of homo sapiens and quadrupeds who are either carnivorous or herbivorous.

The food contains nutrients for energy, proteins, chemicals, minerals and fluids to keep cellular and skeletal structures in peak condition in order to maintain life. As the food is ingested, the digestive juices, enzymes and mucus from the mucous glands are mixed in the bolus of food as it is masticated and deposited in the stomach by glutition. The acids in the stomach break down the food into absorbable units and it is then propelled into the intestines by the peristaltic action of the diaphragm.

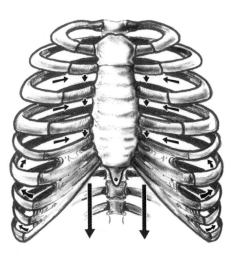

Figure 20: Direction of lymphatic flow of the surrounding muscles of the ribcage.

The intestinal villi, as seen in pathological specimens, draw nutritional requirements for the body out of the bolus of food as it descends through the intestines; the lipid is then drained into the mesenteric lymphatics at the side of the alimentary canal. The enzyme formed in the digastric belly neutralizes the acids in the lipid before it enters the bloodstream. As the mesenteric vessels fill, the portal vein transports the lipid through the portal fissure to pick up hormones, insulin, sodium bicarbonate, blood cells and minerals from glands in the abdominal cavity; the lipid is then pulsated into the liver. Bile pigments, bile salts and alpha amylase, an enzyme produced in glands in the cheeks, fractionize, liquefy and neutralize the lipid, by agitation, to water.

The cardiac cycle pulsates the blood, liquefied nutrients and plasma through the arteries, veins and capillaries, through the fenestrae and into the interstitium for nutrition and maintenance.

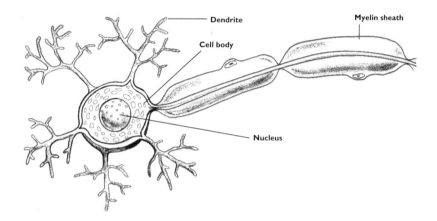

Figure 21: A myelinated nerve fibre capable of sending a nerve impulse at the rate of 80 to 100 metres a second.

Cells

The average tissue cell and contents are listed below:

Lysosomes are involved in the process of localized intracellular digestion.

Mitochondria are small membrane-bounded organelles that are the site of adenosine triphosphate (ATP) synthesis. They also store DNA and RNA plus energy in the form of high-energy phosphate bonds.

Ribosomes are any of the intracellular ribonucleoprotein particles concerned with protein synthesis. They may occur singly or in clusters (polyribosomes).

A *centriole* organelle is located in the *centrosome* (a specialized area of condensed cytoplasm). It is either of two tiny cylindrical organelles in most animal cells that form the poles of the spindle during mitosis (ordinary process of cell division). For further reading, see p1075, *Classic Edition*, 1901 *Gray's Anatomy*. A centrosome is the small mass of differentiated cytoplasm (a complex jelly-like colloidal substance constituting the living matter and performing life functions).

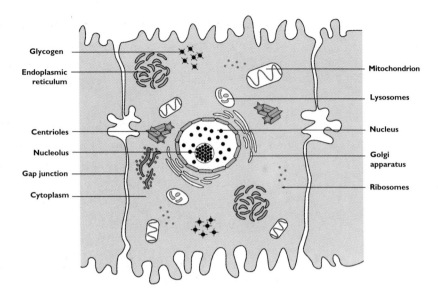

Figure 22: A tissue cell drawn with the cells of digestion within. Numbered and named.

The *cytoplasm* and *protoplasm* of a cell surrounding the nucleus (nucleoplasm) – a complete jelly-like colloidal substance constituting the living matter of plants and animals that surrounds and nourishes the nucleolus within the chromatin.

The *nuclear membrane* surrounding the nucleus and nucleolus filters the nutrients entering from the protoplasm.

The *endoplasmic reticulum* are flattened sacs and tubes, a communicating channel between the nucleus and the cell environment where digestive chemicals are manufactured; also functions in intracellular transport.

Chromatin is a substance of the chromosomes composed of DNA and basic proteins where the new cell is formed in the nucleolus to replace the existing cell at the end of its life. The chromatin within the nucleus splits and releases the new cell. The debris from the expired cell is pulsated by the cardiac cycle into lymphatic vessels to be fractionized, liquefied and neutralized.

The Golgi apparatus is involved in synthesis of glycoproteins, lipoproteins, membrane-bounded protein and lysosomal proteins for digestion and produces the collagenous substance used by the cell to enclose the nutrients as they enter the pits in the cell coat. The sacs are then transported through the cytoplasm to the ribosomes and polyribosomes for digestion. Collagen also encloses the debris from the digestion of nutrients discharged from the ribosomes and polyribosomes in sacs and deposited through the efferent pits in the cell coat into the interstitial fluid for fractionization by the lymphatic system.

The cell membrane (also known as the plasma membrane) differs from other membranes because it bears a diffuse coat of glycoprotein. The cell coat varies from cell to cell and contains sialic acid. It confers on the cell surface an electrostatic charge which is of great importance in the formation of contacts with other cells.

Certain cells live only for a few hours; some live for a few days and others live from one to several months. Their dimensions, as seen under a microscope, are from the size of a small needlepoint (which can be seen with the naked eye) to others which have to be magnified to over 200,000 times to be observed as perfect working spheres within their environment. The above is an overall description of normal cellular and bone functions in animal and plant life.

THE FUNCTIONS OF THE LYMPHATIC, BLOOD AND NERVE SYSTEMS

The Lymphatic System

The lymphatic system is made up of small collecting vessels that have the appearance of a fine wire mesh, like a fly screen. The medial are multidirectional larger vessels containing lymph nodes which form the lymph plexuses and drain the fractionized, liquefied and neutralized "sludge" or fluid into larger, deep blind-ending ducts that propel the fractionized lymph into the large lymphatic glands situated in the abdominal cavity, the inguinals and thorax. The lymph fluid which has been purified to water is then drained into the thoracic duct and subclavian vein into the bloodstream.

These three types of vessel lie in close proximity to the blood vessels and nerve fibres to facilitate the free flow of the nutrition filled blood and the nerve impulse from the brain that innervates all the cellular tissue and bone.

There are between 450 and 500 lymph nodes in the lymphatic apparatus of the human body. Each node possesses fifteen natural killer and agranular cells within its body. At first, I did not believe there was such a high aggregation of cells within the node. However, when visiting the anatomy section of the Adelaide Medical School, I observed an enlarged lymph node in solution, cut in its transverse diameter exposing many more cells within, both natural killer and agranular filtration cells. The agranular cells had the appearance of being filled with a superfine white tapioca seed. I then believed the high aggregation as quoted. I would like to have seen it cut longitudinally, as there could have been more than the cells quoted.

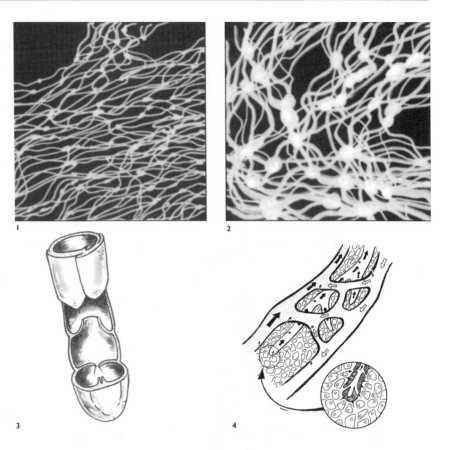

Figure 23: The 3 phases of the lymphatic system in their order: (1) Lymph E the fine vessels that drain the denuded interstitial fluid into the lymphatic system, and: (2) the multidirectional flow that fractionize, liquefy and neutralize the detritus. (3) The deep blind ending valved ducts that transport the purified fluid into the thoracic duct and subclavian veins. (4) A generalized illustration of the interstitial fluid propelled into the interstitium and the overall drainage from the interstitium back into the subclavian veins.

The cells of tissue discharge the metabolic wastes in collagenous sacs into the interstitium. The collagen is produced in the Golgi process of the tissue cells. The effete bone cells are discharged through the epiphyseal ends of bone in a downward flow, which appears to be degenerated to a fine powdery sand. This foreign particulate forms plaques between the joints and is of an abrasive nature (*see* description in arthritis).

The brain discharges the foreign particulate and protein in two ways:

1.   The meningeal lymphatic vessels drain through the same foramina lateral to foramen magnum as the cranial nerves and discharge the meningeal foreign particulate into the deep cervical chains traversing downwards past the cervical vertebrae (*see* figure 23).

2.   The foreign protein from the brain drains through the pons and medulla oblongata of the central nervous system (CNS) and out through the canals of the vertebrae from the cervicals to the coccyx. The detritus from the brain and medulla oblongata is a fatty, waxy, starchy amyloid protein. It

forms plaques in the brain if the draining vessels are blocked and dysfunctional and is the precursor to Alzheimer's disease and dementia. I have also noted amyloid surrounding the vertebral column, which I describe in osteoporosis, from the cranials to the coccyx; the highest aggregation being at the thoracics, 3,4,5 lumbar, sacrum and on the iliac crest.

I have also observed amyloid deposits in the organs – the heart, kidney, spleen, pancreas and liver, which had been cut and in solution at the Adelaide Medical School. It has been observed in the breast, lungs, around the diaphragm and under the skin down to the subcutaneous tissue.

A recent research by scientists from Britain, America and Canada indicated a new vaccine has been developed and tested and is undergoing trials on mice in England. They consider it would probably halt Alzheimer's disease and prevent it spreading. The vaccine attacks the build-up of beta-amyloid, a damaging waxy plaque on the brain cells. They considered it could take another five years before it could be used on humans. This report was printed in the *South Australian Advertiser*, December, 2000.

If the rate of flow of interstitial fluid is below 20 ft/second, patients will be aware of a blocked drainage because the flow is too slow and the gelled plasma and water will not drain through the vessels. The pulsation of the cardiac cycle is not strong enough to propel the foreign particulate and protein through to the deep vessels to be fractionized. The gelled debris has to drain through 8–10 lymph nodes to be fractionized, liquefied and neutralized before it can flow into the subclavian veins. Interstitial fluid is not lymph fluid until it enters the lymphatic system.

The pulsation of the cardiac cycle and propulsion of lymphatic activity is conducted through an airless environment in the body that creates a vacuum. The blood, and the lymphatic fluid and debris, can expand and contract the vessel walls without any problem from the air.

Blood

Blood is a liquid tissue that conveys nutrients, chemicals, minerals, water, plasma, oxygen and warmth through arteries, veins and capillaries pumped by the heart which itself is innervated by the nervous system. The brain receives 30% of the oxygen inhaled from inspiration. The arteries are supplied with blood vessels, nerves and lymphatic vessels within the tunica adventitia, tunica media and tunica intima.

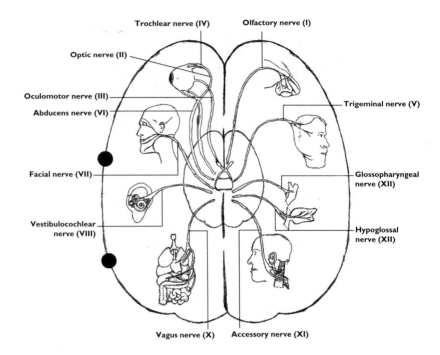

Figure 24: The drainage outlets from the base of the skull that flow into the deep cervicals to the subclavian veins.

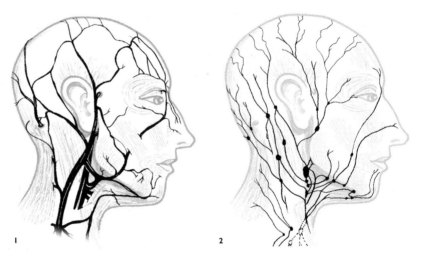

Figure 25: Blood and lymph.
1. Shows the blood flow to the head and brain.
2. This shows the lymph drainage from the head down to the sub-clavian veins.

The veins and capillaries possess fenestrated muscles in their walls. Cardiac innervation expands and contracts the vessels; artery muscles expand longitudinally and do not possess the fenestrae. The fenestrae of the veins and capillaries expand and contract transversely, allowing the interstitial fluid and all nutrients to pass through into the interstitium. As the fluid and nutrients pass through, the muscles act as a sieve and filter out the undigested lipid, blood cells and blood proteins which are retained in the bloodstream. The ingested lipid within the bloodstream is the precursor to cholesterol. The retention of the undigested lipid in the blood is caused by blockage in the downward flow of lymph fluid from the skull and scalp at the temporal bone and ramus. The inhibited drainage at this site fibrillates the nerves of the muscles that surround the digastric glands in the cheeks and digastric belly, and does not produce the enzymes for digestion (i.e. the enzyme alpha amylase that mixes with the bile salts and pigments in the liver inhibiting the conversion of the lipid (a fatty substance) to water). The interstitial fluid does not re-enter the blood vessels from the interstitium.

Relationships of different parts of the nervous systems

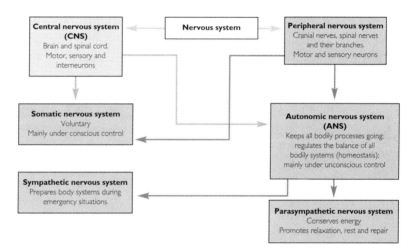

Figure 26: The nervous systems parasympathetic and sympathetic innervating the organs of the body.

Nervous System

The nerve fibres convey an electrical impulse, which is created in the brain by acetylcholine, an acetic acid ester of choline. It is a neurotransmitter at cholinergic synapses and produces the impulse as it crosses the synaptic cleft. An enzyme called acetylcholinesterase catalyzes the action of acetylcholine. Succinylcholine catalyzes both acetylcholine and acetylcholinesterase which clears the synaptic cleft and nerve pathways for the next impulse.

The cranial nerves which arise in the basal ganglia traverse through the foramina of the occipital bone. The central nervous system (CNS) fibres pass through the pons and the medulla oblongata from the diencephalon to the end of the brain stem. The fibres then pass through the cauda equina (peripherals) to the motor end plates of every fibre or flower spray nerve ending.

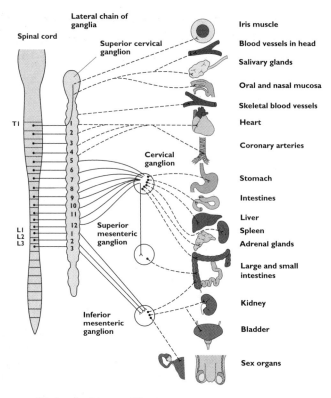

Figure 27: Parasympathetic nervous system.

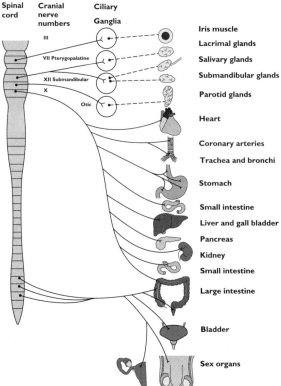

Figure 28: Sympathetic nervous system.

As I work through the striations of muscle fibres, I feel they are innervated and controlled by nerve impulses. They contract the fibres in the belly of the muscle from the centre outwards, towards the origins and insertions in the bone canal. The tension of the annulospinal nerve endings excitate the Golgi nerve end plates to contract and expand. Each nerve end plate controls approximately one hundred fibres.

The above action facilitates the pulsation of the blood within the vessels to flow, and propel the foreign particulate within the lymph vessels past the origins and insertions of fibres in the bone to the deep blind ending valved ducts of the lymphatic system.

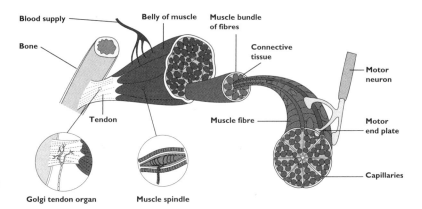

Figure 29: Attachment of muscles to bone and muscle fibre.

The Cardiac Cycle

The central nervous system (CNS) involves the heart and the brain. The brain controls the heart with the chemicals and the thirty-eight hormones it produces, which create the three phases – systole, diastole and diastasis cordis (for further reading see Richard Bergland, *Fabric of Mind*). The brain is the processing centre within the nervous system. The autonomic (involuntary) system stimulates the muscles and glands in the body. Control of the autonomic system is achieved by the two antagonistic – parasympathetic and sympathetic – systems opposing each other.

When the body controls the heart rate, it also controls the flow rate of the blood, interstitial fluid and the lymphatics. Each heartbeat is initiated by a spontaneous discharge within the sinoatrial node – the heart's pacemaker – from the 10th cranial, the vagus, which is a motor and sensory nerve. The rate at which the heart beats is the rate at which the discharges occur. The sympathetic fibres arise from

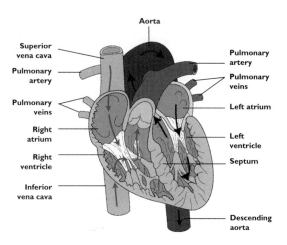

Figure 30: Diagram of heart and blood flow. The heart is innervated by the vagus nerve and controlled by the sympathetic and parasympathetic nerves.

1–5 thoracic nerves and the first 3 segments of the lumbar in the medulla. These fibres excitate and are attached to the heart to boost the heart rate, the smooth muscle and all the glands in the body.

The inhibiting parasympathetic nervous system leaves the CNS with cranial nerves, 3 the oculomotor nerve, (a motor nerve), 7 the facial nerve, (a mixed nerve), 9 the glossopharyngeal (a mixed nerve), and 10 the vagus nerve, (a mixed nerve). The first three are distributed to the heart, a smooth muscle, glands of the head and neck, thoracic abdominal and pelvic viscera. The fibres of the glossopharyngeal are also connected to the vagus nerve.

The secretion of acetylcholine either excites or inhibits certain actions. Acetylcholinesterase cancels out the nerve impulse returning through the dorsal roots of the nerve; succinylcholine cancels out both acetylcholine and acetylcholinesterase before the next spontaneous discharge from the nerve impulse of the cardiac cycle. The balance of their opposing effects determines the rate at which the heart beats.

When you exercise, the heart becomes stretched by the increased flow of blood and other fluids. At times, stretch receptors within the heart chambers initiate impulses that traverse along the afferent (outwards, towards CNS) nerves to a complex of interneurons called a co-ordinating centre in the medulla. This co-ordinating centre responds by increasing the rate at which the impulses are transmitted back to the heart through the sympathetic nerve fibres. This increases the excitatory contribution of the sympathetic synapses, relative to the inhibitory contribution of the parasympathetic synapses, and so increases the heart rate.

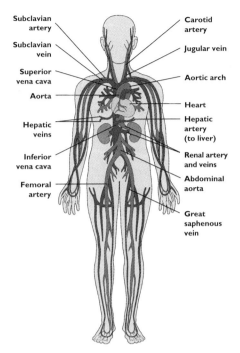

Subclavian artery
Subclavian vein
Superior vena cava
Aorta
Hepatic veins
Inferior vena cava
Femoral artery

Carotid artery
Jugular vein
Aortic arch
Heart
Hepatic artery (to liver)
Renal artery and veins
Abdominal aorta
Great saphenous vein

Figure 31: The cardiovascular system arteries through the body.

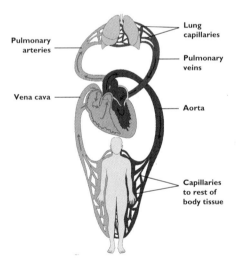

Pulmonary arteries
Vena cava

Lung capillaries
Pulmonary veins
Aorta
Capillaries to rest of body tissue

Figure 32: The circulation system of the body.

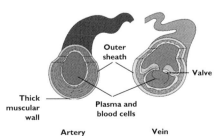

Outer sheath
Thick muscular wall
Plasma and blood cells
Valve

Artery   Vein

Figure 33: Walls of the arteries and veins.

However, what happens when there is a fibrillation of the cranial nerves at the root of the neck and the full impulse from the brain to the sympathetic and parasympathetic synapses is inhibited? An increased level of carbon dioxide in the blood is detected by receptors in the neck arteries. The receptors initiate impulses that travel to the co-ordinating centre and also to cause it to transmit more stimulatory impulses along the sympathetic fibres to the heart, increasing the heart rate.

The above is the way in which the heart is controlled by nerves under normal conditions, but what if the lymphatic system is dysfunctioning through a blockage in any part of the system? This and my earlier question were answered when I worked on the deep lymphatic chains from the cranium to the root of the neck.

Theoretically, the bloodstream should be free of debris, ingested or inhaled, that would contaminate the interstitial fluid that carries nutrients, chemicals and minerals within the interstitium and the deep lymphatic system; capable of propelling the catabolic protein through the vessels, nodes and plexuses to be reduced to water.

Systole is the contraction of the heart muscles, which pulsates the oxygenated blood from the heart cavities. The contraction expands and contracts the arteries, veins and capillaries which pulsate the interstitial fluid containing the water, plasma, nutrients, minerals and chemicals through the fenestrae of the veins and capillaries into the interstitium.

Diastole is the rhythmically occurring relaxation and dilation of the heart atria and ventricles to fill with blood pushed from the veins and capillaries by the pulsation of systole. Diastasis cordis is the rest period to allow the heart cavities to fill before the next systole. Blood, deep lymphatic vessels and nerve fibres lie in close proximity to each other, deep near the bone. The normal heart rate is about 72 to 80 beats per minute, and the rate of flow approximately 20 ft/second.

Part Two

Arrhythmia

I received letters from a patient suffering from arrhythmia. It is described as being an irregular heartbeat or the physiological cycle variations in heart rate, which is related to the vagal impulses to the sinoatrial node. Below is a copy of the letter I sent to 'Joe Smith' in reply:

"Your letter of the 22nd of April is received and noted – thank you. I have asked a lot of questions which have to be taken into account in the assessment and subsequent treatment of your condition, so I will write down the notes I have taken. Yes, I think the lymphatic treatment would help you because it appears to be the same as other heart irregularities.

Have you had any accidents, such as whiplash and/or any other neck/shoulder or back injuries from work, play or sport? Going right back to birth, was it traumatic, such as the use of forceps or other difficult birth procedures; were you an adventurous child, knowing no fear and falling from 'wherever'; playing sport as a teenager and being injured; or at work as an adult – was it trouble-free? All this I take into account before I treat a patient, as any one of the above traumas will cause a similar reaction.

To describe the basic cause, initially I look at the lymphatic system because the practitioner must have a thorough knowledge of anatomy and physiology to know how the body systems work together in harmony.

As I read your letter, I considered your trouble could have started in your early life, because sometimes the heart fibrillation does not manifest until 35–40 years after the basic trauma. You started to feel the effects of 'whatever' two and a half years ago – as you stated, 'short of energy'. Was it short of energy, a general feeling of weakness or lethargy?

1.   Did you have dizzy turns as if you were too weak to move or concentrate?
2.   Did you have an offensive smell in your nose and an offensive taste in your mouth?
3.   Fuzzy heads; not a headache, but a disturbance of some sort, to prevent your eyes focusing correctly?
4.   Out of breath if you tried to hurry and heart palpitations?
5.   Have a tight feeling across your chest at about the 4th –5th rib level?

6.   Muscles and ligaments felt as if they had 'glue' in their fibres? This is the usual procedure of the systems when the heart does not receive the impulse of the nerves that innervate and control its action or beat.

Atrial fibrillation is caused by the dysfunction and/or malfunction of the lymphatic system, whereby it does not clear the pathways of the nerve fibres and blood vessels. The deep blood vessels, lymphatic vessels and nerve fibres lie in close proximity to each other. To describe this condition when it first came to my attention many years ago, I studied each system separately, noting its role in the living bodies of *homo sapiens* and quadrupeds, the effects and affects of each system, if a dysfunction or blockage occurred, and the results healthwise. The next phase I studied was in the direction the body fluids drained. It took me 35 years to find the answer.

As in your atrial fibrillation, the vagus nerve impulse has been fibrillating. The parasympathetic nerves control the heart cycle and the loss of energy or lethargy is the result. In your problem, the first part of the body affected is the neck from the head downwards to the root of the neck. I see a swelling around the root of the neck, above the scapulae, clavicle, thoracic vertebrae and on the cervical, which looks like a horse collar. This is blocking and fibrillating the nerve impulse as it traverses through the nerve fibres from the brain to the motor end plate in the cellular tissue and bone. With the impulse being fibrillated, the force is not strong enough to propel the debris from the interstitial spaces at 20 ft/second from the heart and other organs whereby it gels. The calcium phosphate and calcium then act upon it in our systems, forming an ectopic calcification.

The nerve supply to the heart is through the vagus nerve. It activates the sinoatrial node, Wernicke's fibres, Thorel's bundles, atrioventricular node and Purkingie's fibres. The peripheral nerve system controls the heart beat and sensory nerves send 'information' to the cardioregulatory centre in the medulla.

The heart beat is regulated by the parasympathetic system which slows down the 'racing' heart; the sympathetic nervous system has its roots in the first five thoracic nerves and speeds up the heart beat if it is too slow. If you have atrial fibrillation, the vagus nerve impulse has been fibrillated, the parasympathetic nerves control the heart cycle and the loss of energy or lethargy is the result.

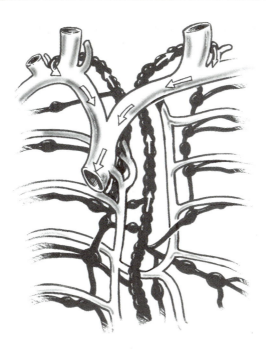

Figure 34: The thoracic duct and blood vessels showing direction of flow.

To treat this and to clear the debris, I use steam heat from hot foments. Wool blankets dipped in boiling water in an old washing machine and wrung out by the wringer attached to the washing machine. Old electric blankets can be used, minus the wiring, which can be pulled out. Microwave ovens can also be used to heat the blankets. Wet the blanket pieces, but do not have the water running out of them. Put in a plastic shopping bag after they are rolled up, and put the bag, tightly rolled, into the microwave on high for 3–5 minutes. Place the pad on the patient's affected area with as much heat as the patient can tolerate. Before heating, put a small hole in the bag before heating to let out steam whilst heating, otherwise the bag might explode.

As in your case, no heart conditions prevail so what is it that medical science cannot diagnose? Do we look at a dysfunctional lymphatic system?

Work flat-handed with as much pressure as the patient can take after the heat application around the neck, over the shoulder, across the chest, up and down the spine, around the ribcage, backwards and forwards on the intercostal muscles between the ribs, but predominantly back towards the spine to push the liquefied debris towards the thoracic duct. Most of this sequence is done while the patient is sitting in a chair. Put the patient prone on the plinth; work flat-handed again. Work up and down the spine and around the ribcage. Put pads on between the massage. Then turn the patient supine and work flat-handed transversely across the abdominal cavity, starting from the diaphragm to work over the spleen, stomach, pancreas, duodenum, jejunum and liver. Work equal pressure transversely over the small intestines (ileum) and colon down to the transtubercular plane.

On each side of the umbilicus in the obliquus muscles, a lymph plexus will be felt under the right and left rectus abdominis, above the omentum. These plexuses are part of the lymphatic chain, draining the oblique muscles. If they are blocked by debris, the nerves from the lumbar and sacrum causes lower back pain described elsewhere.

The drugs you are ingesting are obviously not helping to overcome your arrhythmia. The only thing I know to alleviate the loss of energy is the massage and steam heat as described above."

I saw 'Joe' on the 22nd March, 1999 and gave him a treatment. Heart irregularities non-existent; off all medication and heart back to normal. *Thank you practitioner Katherin Townsend for following the instructions for this patient.*

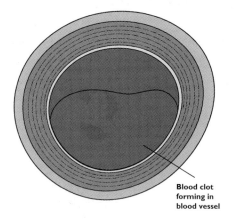

Figure 35: A blood clot forming in a blood vessel.

Blood clot forming in blood vessel

Tom

A few years ago, a friend had an arteriography examination to determine the cause of a suspected slight stroke. A pig's tail catheter was used in the heart and arteries for their investigations. Two slight obstructions were located; one in the carotid artery and the other in the femoral artery. Although the doctor noted the slight obstructions, he did not describe the formation. Nothing else was found in the arteriograph and their description – nothing patent and no abnormalities, particularly in and around the aorta and heart. The medical diagnosis was a 'transient stroke'.

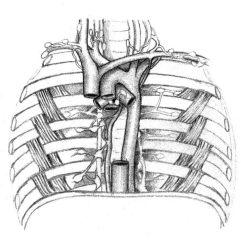

Figure 36: Illustration showing the pathways of the purified lymphatic fluid draining into the subclavian veins. The fluid is pulsated into the heart to liquefy the serous blood which has been drained into the heart chambers.

Normally, the fibrillar obstructions are formed from a fibrinoid thread which occurs naturally in blood. If the blood flow is inhibited, or if a blood vessel is injured, the fibrinoid threads form a barrier at the site of the injury. This repairs the injury in the healing process to prevent blood loss.

Fibrin threads form a clot in an artery or vein when the lymphatic system blockage puts pressure on the nerve fibres inhibiting the nerve impulse from the brain that innervates the blood vessels and slows down the rate of flow of the blood.

I had previously treated this man for an arthritic condition in the arms, shoulders and back. I did not complete the treatment, but gave him sufficient relief from the condition and freedom from pain. He owned a small truck and worked as a private contractor carting goods for large companies. The work involved lifting and carrying cartons, light and heavy; large and small.

As the arteriography examination was in a category concerning heart problems, great care was taken during the physical examination. I, too, found the two obstructions, not in the arteries, but in the lymphatic plexuses adjacent to the arteries.

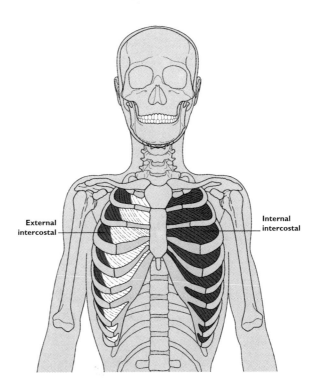

External intercostal

Internal intercostal

Figure 37: The intercostal muscles external and internal. The nerve fibres, blood vessels and lymph vessels are situated between the 2 sets of muscles to flow freely between the ribs.

1.   The carotid obstruction was located in the apical plexus and the lymphocentres of the supraclavicular at the root of the neck. The vagus nerve impulses from the basal ganglia to the heart and lungs were being fibrillated.

2.   The femoral obstruction, not in the artery but in an enlarged inguinal lymph gland situated superior to the pubis and inferior to the inguinal ligament that inserts into the superior iliac spine and pubis. The expansion of this gland put pressure on the artery, nerve and cellular tissue, partially blocking the blood flow and nerve impulse to the leg.

When both blockages were relieved by the work and steam-heated pads, the headaches, dizziness and fibrillation subsided. Full feeling and colour returned to the face, hands and leg.

When the femoral obstruction was relieved by the work described above, the sharp, stabbing pain, locally and in the abdominal cavity at the transtubercular plane reduced in intensity. Warmth and nerve impulses returned to the affected limb and foot.

Arthritis – A Personal View

My husband and I suffered this debilitating disease from 1946, and we were told by our medical advisers to go home, take the prescribed drugs, go to bed until the pain subsided, and order wheelchairs or crutches for mobility, as nothing more could be done for us medically. We had other ideas and began treating ourselves by doing massage and using hot foments to get relief; and we did. Ten weeks later, my husband went back to driving one of the trucks in the fleet we owned, and I went back to doing the farm work.

We were in limbo for a few years as to why we successfully overcame the trauma of this disease. We gained further knowledge as we treated other patients and they had the same relief as we did. As we treated the patients, we gained knowledge of different aspects of the systemic proliferations that presented. Our questions were:

1.   What was it?

2.   What is the basic cause?

The most abundant substance encountered was a fine powdery chalk that appeared to consolidate into a plaque between the joints of the bones and around the insertions/origins of muscle fibres into bone. Again, we asked the questions:

What is it? – From where does this chalky substance that formed the plaque originate? Is it produced from the skeletal or cellular structures, something ingested or inhaled, or from a metabolism, anabolism and catabolism of our diet? Again, no satisfactory answers.

Several years later, our younger daughter went to university and trained as a chiropodist (now referred to as a podiatrist). Her medical books revealed the system most relieved from the massage and steam heat was the lymphatic system. I then checked the other systems in the body, described below, to try and find anything concerning the basic cause of the arthritic problem.

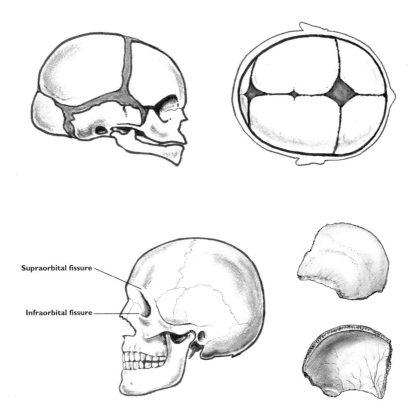

Figure 38: The sutures of bone, the 6 fontanelles, the foraminas, supraorbital and infraorbital fissures and the orebeform plate in the ethmoid bone are all drainages of the brain in adulthood.

Supraorbital fissure

Infraorbital fissure

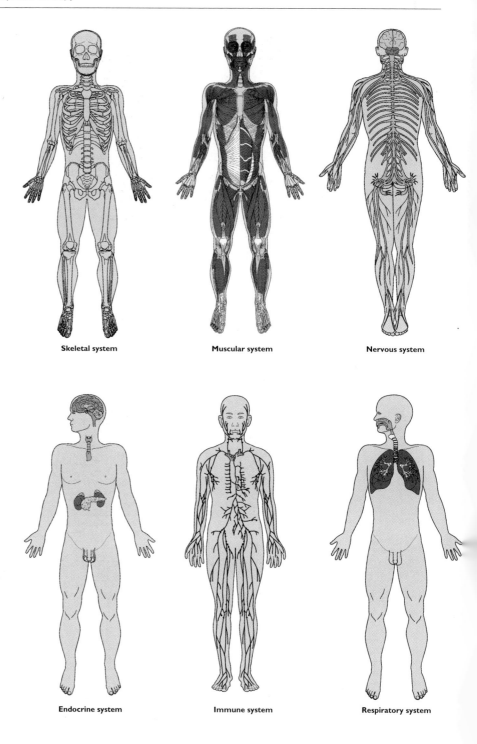

Skeletal system   Muscular system   Nervous system

Endocrine system   Immune system   Respiratory system

Figure 39: All the systems of the body.

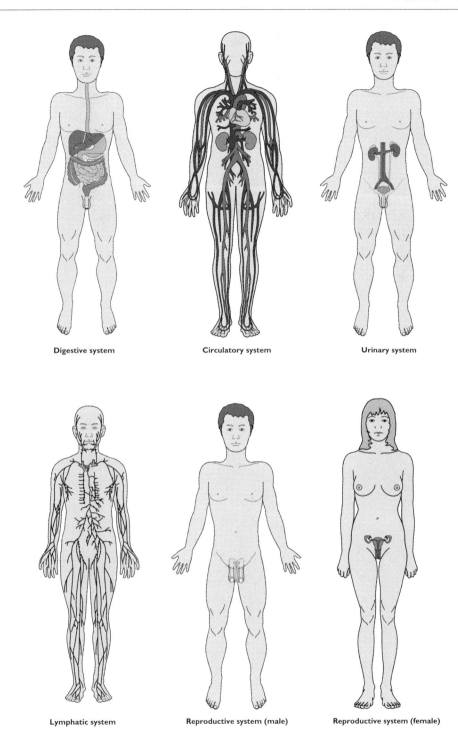

Digestive system

Circulatory system

Urinary system

Lymphatic system

Reproductive system (male)

Reproductive system (female)

Applied Anatomy and Physiology

The integumentary system consists of the skin and its appendages, hair, nails, and sweat and sebaceous glands; it protects deeper tissues from injury. Location of cutaneous pain, pressure and temperature control.

The muscular system refers to all of the muscles of the body, including the smooth, cardiac, and striated muscles, considered as an interrelated structural group.

The skeletal system protects and supports body organs; it provides a framework and attachment for muscles used to cause movement. The bones are a specialized form of intercellular substances which are hardened by calcification.

The nervous system is the fast acting control of the body; responds to internal and external changes by innervating appropriate muscles and glands.

The endocrine system refers to the network of ductless glands and other structures that elaborate and secrete hormones directly into the bloodstream. It regulates processes such as growth, reproduction and nutrition.

The cardiovascular system refers to the blood vessels that transport blood enriched with oxygen, nutrients, minerals and chemicals for skeletal and cellular maintenance. The cardiac cycle – systole, diastole and diastasis cordis – pulsates blood through arteries, veins and capillaries.

The lymphatic system consists of the tissue fluid from the interstitial spaces which is propelled into the valved ducts of the deep lymphatics, transporting all foreign particulate and foreign protein from all the systems in the body; it disposes of the toxic wastes by fractionization, liquefaction and neutralization by the natural killers and filtration cells within the nodes and glands before returning the purified water back into the bloodstream through the subclavian veins.

The respiratory system keeps blood constantly supplied with oxygen and removes carbon dioxide and lactic acid. The gaseous exchanges occur through the pulmonary alveoli, which are surrounded by networks of capillaries through whose walls the exchange of carbon dioxide, lactic acid and oxygen takes place.

Alveolar walls are composed of a single layer of cells and thin boundaries of capillaries, which is all that separates blood and air. Exchanges of the gases across this barrier are completed in a fraction of a second.

The digestive system breaks down food into absorbable units that enter the blood for distribution to cellular tissue and bone. Indigestible foodstuffs and fluids are eliminated from the body as faeces and urine.

The urinary system discharges urine from the kidneys, through the ureters, bladder and urethra and is controlled by several sets of muscles, including the internal and external sphincters. Waste products are eliminated in urine. The urine may also become cloudy from mucus. Persistent cloud may indicate the presence of pus, blood or dead bone cells This has been noted when treating patients with arthritis and osteoporosis.

The overall function of the male/female reproductive systems is the procreation of life. Testes produce sperm and male sex hormones; ducts and glands aid in the delivery of viable sperm to the female reproduction tract. Ovaries produce eggs (ovum) and female sex hormones. The zygote, the cell resulting from fertilization, is known as the embryo until the first trimester (3 months) and thereafter the foetus until full term.

Clinical Considerations in Arthritis

The first symptom I look for in an arthritic patient is the stiffening and distortion of bone joints. This includes inflammation, sensitivity to touch, swelling and heat at the insertions and origins of muscle and ligament fibres into the cortical bone. There is no periostial surface at the attachments of muscle and ligaments in any part of the body. I learnt from both practical work and pathological research that for two reasons the periosteum is absent:

1.   If the muscle fibres are over-exerted, they would tear the periosteum from the bone as do ligaments and tendons if they attach to muscle fibres. The insertion/origin is a drainage for bone debris as it drains from the canals.
2.   There arc other aspects to be considered as to the basic cause from conception to the onset of the 'disease', e.g.:

1. What drugs were administered to the mother, viz. Thalidomide, hormones, etc., during pregnancy?

2. Was embryo/foetus manipulated (turned in utero by medical practitioner) before birth because of breech, back or shoulder presentation?

3. Foetal head engaging in birth canal causing muscle cramp, preventing birth procedures?

4. The above will induce infant's body movements with uterine contractions to rotate on the facets of the occipital and atlas bones while the head is 'locked' in the birth canal.

5. This will cause a 'leak' or seepage of bone protein from the muscles being ruptured by the abnormal movements. The seepage was noted whilst treating an epileptic patient as it had calcified at the base of the occipital and fibrillating the cranial nerves as they emerged from the foramina of the skull.

Nerves, blood and lymphatic vessels lie along the periosteum before entering canals in the bone. These vessels, as observed in animals, are enclosed in a collagenous substance between the muscles to prevent lacerations to their walls. There are also fibrous covered sacs, which possess a mucus secretion between the individual muscles attached in strategic places by fibres to prevent lacerations of the opposing muscle walls as they are activated. Of all the systems in the body, there are only three actively responsible for motivation and maintenance:

1. The blood vascular system;
2. The lymphatic system;
3. The nervous system.

The lymphatic vessels are represented by both small and large vessels, superficial to deep, in musculature and bone, lymph nodes, small and large, singly or in groups, in a plexus or junction. The arthritic condition is located in the epidermis in which the layers (lying in the following order) are:

1. Stratum corneum;
2. Stratum lucidum;
3. Stratum granulosum;
4. Stratum spinosum;
5. Stratum germinativum.

The fine lymphatics appear to be in-between the above layers, which are easily fractionized, liquefied and neutralized to flow through the dermis which is attached to the subcutaneous adipose tissue or superficial fascia. The flow of interstitial fluid is propelled into the deep, valved ducts of the lymphatics, together with all the foreign particulate and protein, by the pulsation of the cardiac cycle. The fluid flow or drainage is multidirectional.

As I work, I note a similarity in all patients. The precursor to the onset of rheumatoid arthritis is caused by: a fall, a blow of some description, playing violent sport, a car or vehicle accident, or anything that would twist and pull muscle and ligament fibres out of the canals in the skeletal structure and rupture the cellular tissue. All of these would cause a leakage of bone protein from the canals.

As the cells rupture, the calcium in the musculature penetrates the cells and enters the mitochondria, mixes with the phosphate bonds which fibrillates the nerve impulse and reduces the rate of flow from 20 ft/second to complete blockage or just a seepage. Blood clots will form, interstitial fluid and lymph will gel and the nerve impulse from the brain to the motor end plates of the nerve fibre is inhibited.

A tissue cell will die if it is more than a micron away from the flow of nutrients, chemicals and minerals in the interstitial fluid. Interstitial fluid, as I see it, would be approximately 50% water and 50% plasma, a product of plasma cells formed in the diaphysis of the trabeculated bone and transported to the bloodstream as required. Any blockage as above, blocking the nutrient canals of the bone, would inhibit the supply of plasma to the bloodstream. The debris from the bone structure – dead bone cells, nutrient debris, effete plasma cells and bone marrow – is discharged from the epiphyseal ends of the bones. When injured in any type of accident and the fluid drainage inhibited, the foreign particulate from the bones, instead of being drained off in the fluid environment by the pulsation of the cardiac cycle, remains within the joints.

I observed this over fifty years ago in animals, and again about twenty years ago in and around the bones of homo sapiens. The foreign particulate stays within the joints and as the patient tries to move, the water in the debris is drained out by the weight of the body. It then leaves the effete bone debris and dead bone cells bound together by the oil content of the plasma to form plaques in-between the opposing bone structures. As the sand/chalk alkaline plaque consolidates in between the joints, the 'sandpaper' effect of the waste wears away the synovial cells that lubricate the joints. When these cells are lost, the plaque then wears away the cartilaginous coat, which protects the cortical and trabecular structure of the bone ends. The bones then fuse together making it necessary for knee joints in particular to be broken under anaesthetic for mobility.

Some animals (sheep) noted years ago were affected right through the cellular tissue and every joint. The collaginous sacs between the muscles to prevent degeneration of the muscle walls were calcified up to the epidermis. My questions when I observed the calcifications, which were not answered for many years were:

1.   What is it? I could not see or find anything in the carcase to indicate its origins.
2.   Why does it appear to be attached to the bone and grow in thin 'sheets' up to the skin?
3.   What causes the gradual build-up of this chalk/sand-like deposit – was it the result of injury or was it something the animal had eaten?
4.   Why did it form the chalk/sand-like substance between the muscles?

About twenty years ago, I saw a patient who could not walk properly without pain. His foot and ankle appeared to be fused together. As he had already arranged with his doctor to have an operation, I only treated him once. After his operation, he showed me the foreign particulate excised from the ankle and foot. I immediately thought of the animals that had experienced the same condition. It was a chalk/sand-like substance – cream/yellow in colour, which had formed plaques between the bones with indentations of a similar shape to the tarsal and cuneiform bones of the foot. I crushed a small portion of the plaque and it reduced to a powder. In its solid form it was bound together by an oily substance, as were the specimens taken from the animals – obviously it was the plasma content of the interstitial fluid. Plasma is an amber-coloured fluid and a light, translucent oil, which mixes with water in the blood, hence the colour of the plaques. After examining the foreign particulate, the plaques were placed in solution in a container and sealed. The patient allowed me to keep these specimens for observation.

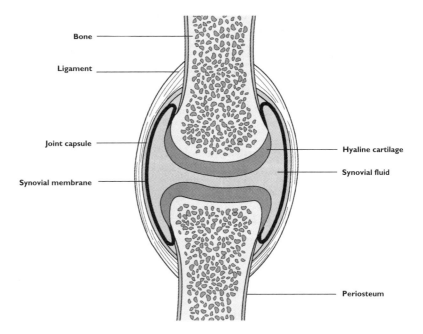

Bone

Ligament

Joint capsule

Synovial membrane

Hyaline cartilage

Synovial fluid

Periosteum

Typical synovial joint

Figure 40: The synovial fluid lubricates the joints.

After a week in the fluid, they disintegrated to smaller pieces; within a fortnight, the smaller pieces degenerated to a cream/yellow 'cloud' in the liquid. At the end of the month, all the solid plaque had liquefied and represented the appearance of a cloudy urine.

The pain from any arthritic condition is excruciating. The acidic chalk / sand-like exudate formed around the deep nerve fibres fibrillates the nerve impulse from the brain to the motor end plates in the cellular tissue and bone. It gives off an acidic burning vibratory pain, the intensity of which paralyzes the patient. If left untreated, the calcium/phosphate combination will form brittle bone plaques at any of the joints. As the plaque debris increases in volume within the body structures, the cellular tissues develop a pale green/yellow translucency – with it a 'pins and needles' sensation as the complaint advances through the intramembranous and endochondral types of bone.

When X-rays or scans are taken to determine the cause and effect of the complaint described, all that can be seen is the distortion of joints and a white 'cloud' obliterating the musculature. Some call it ectopic and others call it a dystrophic calcification. To treat, I do not find any difference in the above classifications as they both respond equally to treatment.

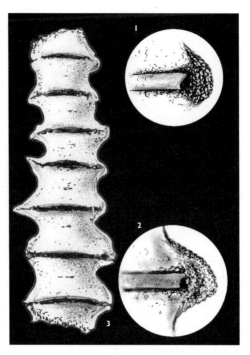

Figure 41:
{ 1. The fine
{ 2. collecting ducts.
3. Calcification of a spine.

My observation of the fluid drainage and subsequent research proved the debris that emerged from the epiphyseal ends of bone would be drained in an upward or downward flow of the interstitial fluid and propelled into the deep valved ducts of the lymphatics by the pulsation of the cardiac cycle. I found that as I worked on the muscles and the collagenous sacs, I released the foreign particulate that was calcifying the mucus secretion within. I applied steam heat on the particulate in the body and the plasma, which had gelled within the cellular blockage, would seep out and drain off in the direction of flow as it liquefied. The rate of flow would escalate as I massaged flat-handed in the direction of flow; the increased pressure of the interstitial fluid pulsated into the interstitium, plus the liquefaction of the gelled debris would 'wash' the outer part of the blockage.

I requested patients to tell me if, by the removal of the above debris, it would feel as if I was pushing something too solid into vessels that were too small to cope as they are only the size of a human hair. The answer was invariably affirmative. However, I was already aware of this, as I had experienced the same problem when being treated for my own arthritic condition.

I use a lot of steam heat in treating arthritis because it liquefies the gelled plasma, even in the debris that is calcifying into brittle bone. It fractionizes into a coarse sand and as it begins to move with the specialized massage, the steam heat liquefies the exudate to a watery consistency. This allows it to flow into the lymph nodes where the natural killer cells and agranular filtration cells within neutralize the water before it enters the bloodstream at the subclavian veins. I observed the cells within the lymph node, in a specimen in solution at the Medical School in Adelaide.

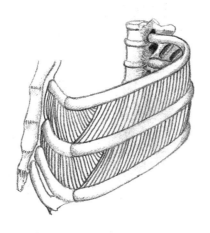

Figure 42: Diaphragm discharges fluid into the inframammary plexus. Fluid drains under the breast upwards. It also drains between intercostal muscles between the ribcage, back into the thoracic duct.

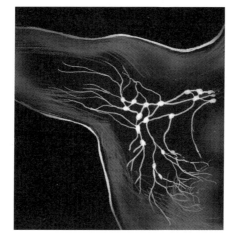

Figure 43: The deep plexuses drain the fluid from the diaphragm and the breast into the subclavian vein. If there is an excess of fluid it will flow transversely to the parasternal nodes; it then flows downward under the rectus abdominis and over the omentum to the plexuses lateral to umbilicus. From there it drains over pubis and into the perineum.

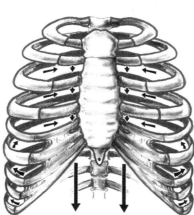

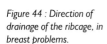

Figure 44 : Direction of drainage of the ribcage, in breast problems.

Breast Problems

The human breasts are situated on the 3rd–7th ribs from near the sternum to near the axilla. They lie over the pectoral muscles and are separated from them by a layer of fascia. The nipple is surrounded by the areolar, a tissue containing small spaces as well as sebaceous glands that contain a fatty secretion for lubrication. Within the breasts are milk-secreting lobes and lobules connected by areolar tissue, blood, lymphatic vessels and lactiferous ducts. The arteries within come from the thoracic, intercostal and internal mammary branches. Veins and lymphatic vessels surround the nipple; the blood drains into the axillary and internal mammary veins.

The lymphatic vessels, devoid of lymph nodes within the breasts, drain from the nipple out and downward towards the plexuses named, within its circumference:

1. The inframammary plexus, situated inferior and lateral to the breast and medially towards the sternum, drains the fine vessels situated in the breast laterally and upward to the axillary plexus. The lymph fluid drains posteriorly from the fine vessels into the intercostals in the ribcage into the multidirectional and deep blind-ending valved ducts to the thoracic duct.

2. The parasternals medially also drain the fine vessels of the breasts. The lymph then drains inferiorly past the xiphoid process and under the rectus abdominis above the omentum towards the linea alba into the plexuses lateral to umbilicus. The drainage from the lateral umbilical plexuses and omentum is felt by the patient to converge to three vessels: two large vessels draining around the pubic bone and another vessel draining under linea alba into and around symphysis pubis. The drainage below this point will be described elsewhere.

3. The drainage from the deep scapula plexus near teres major, teres minor and the deep axillary end nodes flows in two directions. Firstly under and over scapula towards the root of the neck through thestriations of the muscle fibres of trapezius, rhomboids and serratus posterior. Secondly from the axillary plexus and deep under scapula into the central group and subclavian before entering the apical group of vessels and nodes.

4. The drainage from the fine vessels in the breasts flows into the lateral deep vessels of the brachial and intermediate plexuses. From there it drains into the infraclavicular plexus and finally into the subclavian vein.

5. The supraclavicular plexus drains from the root of the neck near the apical group to the infraclavicular plexus which are superior and inferior to the clavicle into the subclavian vein.

6. The deep cervical chains drain from the bony labyrinth of the occipital bone, between the spinous process and transverse spines of the vertebrae down to the filum terminale.

7. If the vessels close to the infraclavicular plexus are blocked, the mammary plexus surrounding the lateral and superior part of the breast will drain the lymph fluid across the ribcage into the parasternals from the fine vessels in the breasts. If the above blockage occurs, lumps of detritus are felt in the fine vessels of the breasts, the precursor to growths, benign or malignant (*see* page 77, head and shoulder drainage).

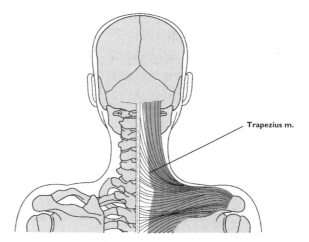

Trapezius m.

Figure 45: The trapezius muscles.

The lymphatic vessels within the breast are devoid of lymph nodes for obvious reasons that if the lymph nodes are blocked, at or after the birth of offspring, the foreign particulate within the blocked drainage would release foreign protein into the lacteals as it decomposed. The principle would be identical to a mother breast feeding the baby with silicon implants embedded in and around the lacteals. One such case was advertised in one of the popular women's magazines in recent years. The mother gave birth but did not have the implants removed. The baby ingested the silicon from the implants, became very ill and was not expected to live! A breast has a 360° drainage from the nipple, areola and lacteals into the plexuses named in the previous section, numbered 1–7.

If tight underwear, particularly underwired bras, are worn the pressure from the wire and the hard padding surrounding the wire puts pressure on the plexuses listed and prevents the propelled drainage from the breast to the medial multidirectional flow from being fractionized, liquefied and neutralized. The tight garment prevents free drainage and holds the lymph and interstitial fluid within the breast tissue and lacteals. The plasma and waste form a gel which consolidates into a benign growth when the flow is slowed down by the blockage. The benign growth then sends a micro-organism aerobe into the healthy cells adjacent to the growth to ingest the oxygen within the cells which causes death. The foreign protein produced by anaerobic fractionization enters the benign growth which then accelerates in size to form a malignancy.

I received a message recently from a patient in England who had treatment in Gloucestershire for lumps in her breast. She stated: "I feel a lot better from having the lymphatic drainage from you and Jenny. Many thanks. Look forward to seeing you again in the New Year."

The massage must be light and flat-handed around the base of the breast and on the ribcage where the blockage occurs as a seepage instead of a full drainage into the multidirectional vessels. Steam heat must be used to liquefy the foreign particulate because the foreign particles will only move to another site, overloading the nodes in the plexuses, and form another malignancy.

I have noted for many years that I have not been able to do effleurage, rolfing and hacking in DLT. Effleurage is very soothing because of the gentle use of hand movements from the wrist, massaging with the palm and heel of the hand with stroking movements of the fingers. It does not penetrate between the muscles and ligament to innervate the three phases of the lymphatic system. This has to be demonstrated.

Rolfing and hacking will only give a slight relief to the fine phase in the movement of the vessels under the dermis and epidermis but will consolidate any blockage in the second and third phase. Flat hand, straight finger movement between the muscles and ligaments down to the bone must be used to remove any blockage in the deep vessels' direction of flow. Again, this must be demonstrated.

To treat a patient with lymphatic dysfunction within the fine drainage vessels and plexuses I firstly sit them in a chair, lightly massage around the head, neck, shoulders, ribcage and spine working flat-handed. If necessary, hot steam-heated pads are applied while in the chair to liquefy the gelled interstitial fluid and debris. The liquefied debris will be integrated with the interstitial fluid pulsated into the interstitium by the cardiac cycle and facilitate the drainage into the deep vessels.

I do not work on the breast or any obstructions or growths, benign or malignant, until the plexuses can drain the liquefied debris in sufficient quantity to prevent an 'overload' and blockage in another part of the system. Once drainage has been initiated, the lymph nodes are activated. The fifteen natural killer and agranular filtration cells within the node will again fractionize, liquefy and neutralize the 'rogue' cells within the obstructions. A 'rogue' cell only goes through 8 or 10 lymph nodes to be purified to water.

There is an exception to the rule with breast obstructions. I recently treated a patient whose breast was discoloured. It was red/purple in colour and had a large obstruction under the nipple and in the surrounding glands.

I held the breast with one hand and very lightly massaged around the nipple, areola and breast with the other hand working very lightly, flat-handed, circling the breasts. I used a lot of steam heat whilst I massaged.

Hematomas are easier to treat than an ordinary growth or obstruction because the steam heat liquefies the coagulum. The hematoma in this case was the size of a small hen's egg that had been boiled and cut longitudinally. After the first treatment I could feel the coagulum liquefying. By the fourth treatment there was only a quarter of the obstruction remaining.

When treating a patient recently with diagnosed melanoma, I observed the blocked lymphatic drainage from the operation and two radiotherapy treatments performed last year.

The right breast had not been excised but there was a deep scar on the lateral side from the areola to the ribcage. It was adjacent to other deep scars where the pectoral muscles, together with the mammary, axillary, brachial, intermediate and subclavian plexuses had been excised. Scar and discolouration of tissues were evident where the radiotherapy had been performed. Nerve fibres, blood vessels and all fluid drainage had been cut or blocked.

From the 5th–8th ribs raised lesions anteriorly, as hard as bone and a purple colour, at the superior aspect of the breast had formed, too painful to touch by hand or to wear even loose clothing. The patient was ingesting morphine twice a day to control the pain. The operation scars where muscles and drainage vessels had been removed under the arm down to the bone were puckered where the skin had been stitched.

A hard lesion, the size of a walnut, was situated at the edge of where the axillary nodes had been removed and near the teres major and teres minor muscles. It was extremely painful to touch and the patient could not lie on her right side when in bed. She was told that it was a melanoma cancer, as all the lesions were hard.

Pain extended through the right side to trapezius, rhomboideus major and minor, through to ligamentum nuchae, extending to the muscles on the left shoulder.

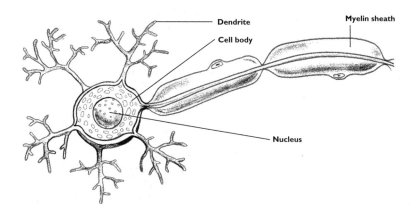

Figure 46:

The phrenic nerve, which arises from the 2nd cervical nerve and is attached to all cervical nerves to the root of the neck, had either been cut or burnt from the radiotherapy and was not functioning. Its innervation is from the cervical nerves as above and it traverses deep into the mediastinum, down to the root of the lung, through the bottom lobe and is attached to the diaphragm. The left branch innervates the left lung and part of the pericardium and the left side of the diaphragm. The right branch innervates the right lung and the right side of the diaphragm.

If a fibrillation occurs, left or right, both sides of the diaphragm do not co-ordinate to initiate the peristaltic action on the organs and glands in the abdominal cavity, or to innervate the lungs for inspiration/expiration. If peristaltic action is absent, constipation occurs, as with this patient; her bowel had blocked for 18 days before medical intervention.

The innervation of the lungs discharges the gases and fluid from the pulmonary alveoli. Again, if peristaltic action is inhibited, the fluid content in the lungs is not expired and accumulates in the pulmonary alveoli. The patient, by medical intervention, finally had 14 pints of fluid aspirated from the lungs in 24 hours, otherwise she would have 'drowned' in her own fluid.

When I first treated the patient, I did four treatments a day for the first two days using only hot foments and very light massage. At the third day I reduced the treatments to once a day because the fine lymphatic vessels were reacting by starting to drain the detritus from the area burnt by the radiotherapy.

At this stage I was able to sit the patient upright and work around the walnut-sized obstruction, scapula, and the muscles and ligaments controlling the action of the arm and shoulder.

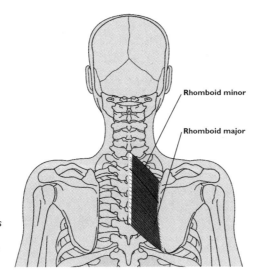

Figure 47: The rhomboid muscles protect the fluid vessels and nerve fibres; they also stabilize muscular action of the shoulder.

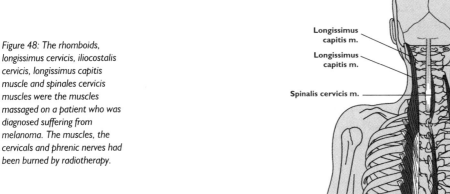

Figure 48: The rhomboids, longissimus cervicis, iliocostalis cervicis, longissimus capitis muscle and spinales cervicis muscles were the muscles massaged on a patient who was diagnosed suffering from melanoma. The muscles, the cervicals and phrenic nerves had been burned by radiotherapy.

At first, just to touch the muscles caused excruciating pain so I only performed a short treatment. Even at the first short treatment the purple colour receded from the growth. At the second treatment the obstruction developed a groove in the centre and the purple colour had disappeared. By the third treatment, the obstruction had split to the extent that I could feel the anterior was a hard nodule, approximately the size of a broad bean. At the fourth treatment I could feel the nodule had disintegrated into two sections, the anterior still a hard nodule and the posterior a multidirectional bundle of vessels that was attached to the hard nodule by one of the larger vessels from the bundle.

One or two days later the upward drainage from the small plexus that had been reactivated drained through the striations of the trapezius and rhomboids to the spine. The root of the neck was blocked on the right side and the 'overload' of fluid from the small plexus had drained into the left side and blocked all the deep cervical chains and plexuses in the left side down to the infraclavicular plexuses. My questions regarding the above are:

1.   Was the growth/obstruction quoted by the patient's specialist a melanoma, or;

2.   Was it an axillary node not excised, blocking part of the lymphatic apparatus that drains the subscapular plexus vessels over and under the scapula?

I did not complete treatment because of the blocked bowel and fluid in the lungs. Too many nerves were fibrillated and the patient could not be helped.

Drainage from Head to Shoulder

Basically, the dysfunction of the drainage is caused by blockage of the drainage from the top of the head downward to the root of the neck. If the patient has an accident and the skull sustains an injury, whiplash, or a rupture of tissue cells as the muscle fibres are pulled from the canals of bone or are damaged by a blow, calcium from the tissue fluid will seep into the damaged cells and mix with the phosphate bonds to create a calcification. The upward drainage towards the subclavian vein from the plexuses surrounding the breasts will be inhibited by the

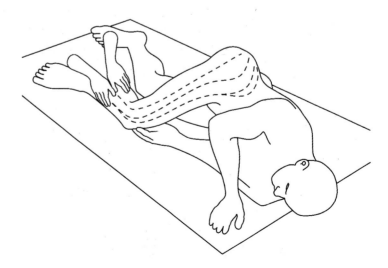

Figure 49: Position of patient on plinth for treatment on lower back pain and male / female body dysfunction.

drainage from the head and neck. The rate of flow is blocked, the water and plasma in the interstitial fluid gels, and the calcium and phosphate bonds calcify. The debris held in the body at 98.4°F will degenerate and produce the micro-organism aerobe and the enzyme anaerobe. The aerobe ingests the oxygen from the healthy cells, which then die.

The anaerobe fractionizes the dead cells to cause a malignancy. This is the main reason for not working through an obstruction or blockage because the debris is too thick to flow freely through the natural killer and agranular cells of the lymph nodes and plexuses (*see* page 69, breast problems).

Female

The drainage downward through the umbilical plexuses into the inguinals and into the symphysis pubis will have the same reaction as the drainage from the head. With the female, the fluid is supposed to flow around the clitoris, under labium majora and minora, around Bartholin's glands and into the perineum between the clitoris and vagina. If there is an 'overload' of fluid to enter the perineum, the excess fluid will drain through the obturator foramen and fibrillate the obturator, femoral, saphenous nerves and the twigs and branches of the sciatic nerves. The patient will feel pain in the roots of the adductor magnus muscle down to the knee. From the knee downwards it feels as if a solid wedge is moving and is very painful as it drains into the toes and back to the perineum.

Male

In the body of the male, the drainage is the same as the female to the pubic bone. The flow goes around symphysis pubis. The drainage is painful for both sexes. The fluid flows around the penis, under the scrotum and in vessels in close proximity to vas deferens, epididymis, prostate, urethra and bladder, and finally into the glands below cisterna chyli and thoracic duct. If the drainage is in excess to capacity the fluid traverses downward in the same vessels as the female and again upward to the perineum. The patient will have considerable pain until the fluid pressure subsides.

To treat the above dysfunction, the patient is treated by flat-hand massage, prone and supine, and with the steam-heated foments. I then put the patient, both male and female, on their side, the leg on the upward side bent at the knee on a pillow and the other leg straight. I work between the muscles down to the bone, anterior and posterior to trochanter, up to the roots of the gluteal muscles on the ischium and ilium.

Case Study – Jo

A friend noting 'lumps' in both breasts went to a cancer specialist in the city. He presented her with a form for her to sign to give him permission to perform a mastectomy to remove both breasts, as he considered the growths were malignant. She refused to sign the form and told him she wanted to try alternative treatments first.

He consented to the request and gave her a month to try other treatments. If the growths were still evident he would have to operate; he measured the size of the growths. We started treatment immediately. I gave treatment three times a week and she worked in between.

Three weeks later we were confident there was nothing left of the 'malignancies'. Jo kept her appointment after four weeks and the specialist tried to measure the growths and was very surprised there was nothing left. His only comment was: "We cannot take any notice of this treatment, as it was not done by a medical practitioner."

Twenty years later she still has both breasts and no sign of the cancer! We worked around the breasts on the deep lymphatics, used steam-heated pads and the 'growths' degenerated.

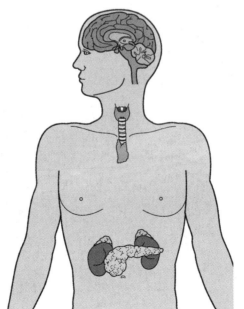

Figure 50: The glands and organs treated for diabetes mellitus.

Diabetes Mellitus

Whilst working on the abdominal cavity of an osteomyelitic patient using flat-hand, transverse massage, coupled with steam heat, he developed diabetes. He visited his doctor, who diagnosed the disorder and put him on a strict diet as his blood sugar level was up to 18.8. I worked on the ribcage and diaphragm and after the first treatment in July, the blood glucose count dropped to 11.8.

When I first studied the digestive system, I noted it relies upon the production of chemicals and enzymes to break down the solid foods ingested. When the aforementioned patient first presented, he had a 'pouch' formation under the mandible, around the throat and neck, the cheeks and root of the neck. It was obvious the salivary and digestive glands did not produce the necessary chemicals, minerals and other products necessary to digest food.

The materials digested in the oesophagus, stomach and liver are drawn out of the intestinal tract by the villi and transported into the mesenteric lymphatic vessels as a lipid. When the mesenteric vessels fill, the lipid is transported by the portal vein through the porta hepatis. Then ducts from the spleen, pancreas, duodenum and jejunum empty their contents into the vein to assist digestion by the agitation of bile salts, bile pigments and alpha amylase. This reduces the lipids and contents to water.

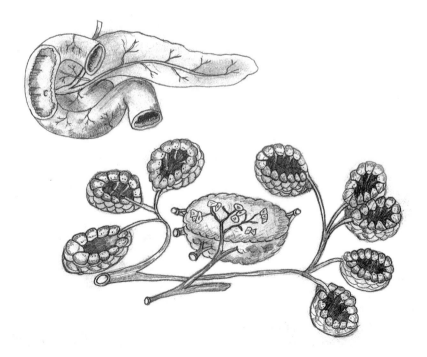

Figure 51: The islets of Langerhans situated in the pancreas, an enlarged view, where work is performed in diabetes mellitus. Work must be performed on the posterior and anterior aspect of the abdominal cavity to release the lymphatic blockage that is preventing the pancreas producing glucagon, insulin and somotostatin.

The pancreas possesses both exocrine and endocrine tissue. The acini (lobes of a gland) secrete digestive enzymes and small ductules secrete sodium bicarbonate solution. The islets of Langerhans, alpha, beta and delta, produce glucagon, insulin and somatostatin, a hormone that controls glucagon and insulin output, in that order. The pancreatic juice enters a long pancreatic duct where it is transported to the duodenum. The bicarbonate ions are both hormonal and neural. The hormone secretions are regulated by the hormone secretin which is an intestinal hormone that stimulates the pancreas to secrete cholesystokinin – a polypeptide hormone – in the small intestine (ileum) to assist gall bladder contraction and secretion of pancreatic enzymes.

The entry of chyme (lipid), which is discharged from the pylorus into the duodenum, transforms proenzyme to prosecretin and into an active secretin, which is released from the mucosa in the top of the duodenum. Mucosa is produced from the mucous membrane that protects the inner lining of the stomach and intestines from destruction by the acids formed in the stomach to break down the food ingested. The partly digested food influences the amount of each hormone released and represents the characteristics of pancreatic juice and alpha amylase, that is secreted in the salivary glands, pancreatic amylase and intestinal amylase, which acts on the starches ingested and reduces it to maltose and isomaltose.

Not anywhere in any report on research, medical books, or any other publication do I find the basic cause of diabetes. My questions were:

1.   What is it?
2.   What is the basic cause of the digestive system failing to break down the sugars and starches, or producing bicarbonate, an alkali? I first worked on the abdominal cavity, over the ribcage, where a large swelling was evident, and the diaphragm. This first treatment reduced the blood sugar level from 18.8 to 11.8. Again, why?

I then remembered my observations in the pathology section of the medical school that I attended where the various organs were strategically placed for maximum output. The pancreas lies transversely behind, slightly inferior to the stomach and between the spleen and duodenum.

When the patient first presented, he had what appeared to be a high concentration of either fluid of a thin collagenous substance in a 'pouch' under and around the mandible, up on to the cheeks to the zygomatic bone and temporal arch, with a blotchy red colour in the skin. At the root of the neck, another swelling appeared, encircling the tissues, lymph plexuses and blocking the fluid vessels. A much larger swelling had manifested on the lower part of the ribcage over the diaphragm, liver, stomach, pancreas, spleen, the transverse colon and ileum. To treat this condition I used a gentle flat hand massage, working transversely with a lot of steam heat. Questions and observations:

1. Was it lymphatic dysfunction because of the high concentration of fluid in the interstitium?

2. The fluid appeared to be half water and half plasma in the dysfunctioning vessels. If a leakage of fluid came through the skin it contained a small amount of oil; the combination of the two fluids will gel if the rate of flow is reduced. By using the hot foments and massage, the gel will liquefy and drain in the direction of flow.

3. I have also noted during massage that there is an increase in the number of nodes and vessels surrounding the digestive glands, plexuses, thorax and diaphragm to fractionize, liquefy and neutralize any gelled particulate that might be detrimental to the wellbeing of the body.

The omentum is also a drainage system from the diaphragm anteriorly down to the transtubercular plane. Vessels from the lower part of the omentum are easily located as they join the upward flow to the legs into the perineum. If there is an excess of interstitial fluid with the toxic debris, other vessels will drain the fluid down the leg medially. This will go through the striations of the adductor magnus muscle fibres and the origins, down through the posterior fibres of the ischial tuberosity, into the anterior fibres from the ramus of ischium and pubis. The patient will note this drainage flow, because the excess toxins and fluid will fibrillate and numb the fibres to the extent that there is no feeling or power in the muscles from the origins down to the knee.

The peristaltic action of the diaphragm on the intestines and linings did not function. The drainage from the cloverleaf formation in the centre of the musculature goes through the striations of fibres of the crural muscles back to the drainage vessels entering the thoracic duct. The muscle fibres surrounding the cloverleaf drain outward and upward over the ribcage into the inframammary plexus and axillary nodes.

As the gelled interstitial fluid and lymphatic particulate had been liquefied and drained, I noted a deep obstruction surrounding the portal, mesenteric and splenic veins. Combined with the liquefied fluids and plasma, the obstruction had the potential to block the release of the digestive juices. This included enzymes, pancreatic amylase, insulin hormones and alkalis from the pancreas, spleen and duodenum into the bloodstream, through the hepatic vein, and being pulsated through the body by the cardiac cycle.

Because of the blocked drainage, the patient became diabetic. As I worked with slow and gentle flat-hand massage transversely, the pain level at first was high at the ribcage and diaphragm. The blood glucose level dropped and the swelling reduced in size. I did not take much notice of the sugar level being lowered and the reduction of the swelling until I treated another patient with an identical problem. One patient dropped from 18.8 to 11.8 and the other patient dropped 10 in blood sugar level in the first treatment. I then did more research on diabetes, both in study and practice. I did not find any reference in any publication or report as to why a diabetic patient's sugar level should drop when the deep lymphatic therapy was practised. Or why the two patients in question (and many others in earlier years of treatment) all went back to normal level of blood sugar, between 4 and 7, without the use of drugs. My conclusions were:

1.   The swelling would have been caused by the retention of interstitial fluid, part calcified or gelled, in the interstitium surrounding the digestive organs and glands, therefore reducing the flow of the interstitial fluid and lymph fluid in the deep lymphatics of the omentum and those surrounding the thoracic duct.

2.   The pressure from the degraded fluid in its gelled form would have restricted the action both anterior and posterior to the islets of Langerhans in the pancreas to reduce production of glucagon, insulin and somatostatin to break down the sugars and starches contained in the diet.

3.   The high pressure of the fluid retention in the interstitium would have inhibited the peristaltic action of the oesophagus and diaphragm.

Blood sugar level of patient in 1997

Early June, at hospital   18.8

Early July, at Diabetes Association   11.8

Early August   10.7

20th August8.1

21st August, before breakfast   6.7

Doctor suggested normal blood sugar level between 4 and 7.

End August 8.2

2nd September   6.5

November   4.0

Patient's blood sugar level has remained at 4 since the last test to the present year.

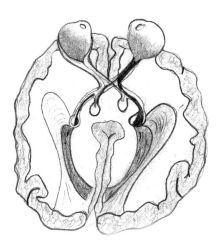

Figure 52: Pathways of left and right optic nerve to the eyes.

Eye Treatment

Muscles of the Eye and Tarsus

Tarsus (pl. tarsi). Any one of the plates of cartilage about 2.5cms long forming the eyelids. One tarsus shapes each eyelid. The levator palpebrae superioris muscle controls the tarsal cartilage.

Inferior oblique – slanting inclined – muscles relaxed would roll eye clockwise or anti-clockwise (as noted in Bell's Palsy).

The optic nerve possesses 1,200,000 fibres. Herman Snellen, a 19th century opthalmologist, devised the testing chart, as seen today, that patients read from a distance of 20 feet.

Muscles Controlling the Eye

Obliquus superior   – innervated by IV trochlear nerve. (4)
Pulls the eye down and outward.

Obliquus inferior   – innervated by III oculomotor nerve. (3)
Pulls eye upward and outward.

Rectus inferior   – innervated by III oculomotor nerve. (3)
Pulls eye downward and inward.

Rectus lateralis   – innervated by VI abducent nerve. (6)
Pulls eye outward.

Rectus medialis   – innervated by III oculomotor nerve. (3)
Pulls eye inward.

Rectus superior   – innervated by III oculomotor nerve. (3)
Pulls eye upward and inward.

The aqueous (or vitreous) humour is a colloid, gelatinous substance that contains nutrients to feed both the cornea and lens. The ciliary body, behind the iris, secretes the aqueous fluid, about a fifth of an ounce a day.

From the ciliary body, the fluid flows into the posterior chamber and then slowly circulates over the rim of the iris towards the pupil and into the anterior chamber behind the cornea. The trabecular meshwork, a webbing of tiny fibres and canals, drains the aqueous humour out of the eye. If these canals are blocked by inadequate lymph drainage, the acidic debris will, in time, damage the nerve fibres that transmit impulses to the peripheral vision because of the fibrillation. The nerves do not die. When the pressure of fibrillation is relieved, the impulse will again traverse the nerve fibres to the motor end plates that innervate the eye muscles. In all the information on eye function and 'cures' from examinations and tests on the eyes for loss of sight, nothing is mentioned of the above or deep lymphatic drainage.

Interstitial fluid is propelled into and through the eye apparatus by the cardiac cycle. The muscles of the eye within the orbit are subject to the same deep lymphatic drainage as the muscles in any other part of the anatomy. Wherever there is a blood vessel, nerve or muscle fibre, a lymphatic vessel, node or plexus is in close proximity. As I treat patients with eye dysfunctions, I observe the following:

1. Zig-zag 'flashes' around the periphery of the eye, which will be similar to a mild electric shock. At the onset, it will bring on a blue-grey 'shadow' of objects before the 'flash'. The muscle action controlling the eye in the orbit will feel as if they are pulling through a glue-like substance – colloidin – a gel-like principle produced in colloidal degeneration. Not much pain produced, but more a feeling of discomfort.

2. The cardiac expansion and contraction of vessels creates a pain (or an eye ache) as fluid that appears to be 'syrupy' is forced through the vessels of the eyeball.

3. A complete opacity of a blue-grey film over the retina, iris and lens in the eye that blocks out all sight.

4. Black dots and squiggles, floating in the aqueous humour as the eye moves.

5. A burning, stinging, itching sensation, noted at times as the eyeballs' drainage canals and tear ducts are blocked with the wastes of metabolism and an excess of acids.

To relieve the above symptoms, I work gently, flat-handed, over the orbit of the eye with a push and pull gliding movement on the lymph vessels and glands. This action causes some tension and the patient can feel fluid movement in the eye. When this occurs, I use hot foments which, with the massage, liquefies the colloidin in the eye, orbit and glands. The fluid then flows out of the eye in copious amounts like sticky tears.

The deep lymphatics within the eye, the iris, around the lens and retina, flow back towards the sutures of the orbit. The fluids and the contaminants drain from the eyeball obliquely towards the pharyngeal, palatine and lingual tonsils and the large nodes in the deep cervical chain, into the plexuses at the root of the neck and then into the subclavian vein.

As mentioned earlier, the interstitial fluid is pulsated into the eye by the cardiac cycle. As it exerts pressure on the fluid content of the body, the fluid is propelled into the deep blind ending lymph ducts at about 6 propulsions a minute.

The interstitial fluid is not lymph fluid until it is propelled into the lymph vessels. If the interstitial fluid is slowed down in the drainage to below 20 feet per second, it will form a gel and block the drainage outlets. It will finally form an ectopic or dystrophic calcification when the calcium in the tissues and the phosphates in the mitochondrion cells of the cellular tissue combines.

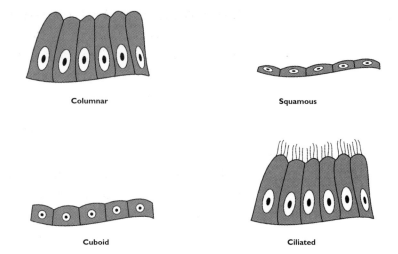

Columnar

Squamous

Cuboid

Ciliated

Figure 53: Epithelial tissue cells.

As I treat patients' eyes by massage, I note that after a few treatments, the iris and pupil, instead of being a natural colour, develop an opacity that looks like a grey 'cloud' permeating the eye. Obviously, I had moved the acidic foreign particulate from the back of the orbit into the aqueous humour where it was liquefied sufficiently to flow through the liquid channels.

A feeling of light headedness accompanied by dizzy spells follow the drainage of the foreign particulate from the eye because of the relief from pressure on the cranial nerves and the release of the acidic wastes. The epithelial coat of the nerve fibres takes from 12 to 36 hours to heal after the above drainage.

I treated a patient in Australia whose sight had regenerated. Initially, his peripheral sight returned, and the photoreceptors improved to the extent that he could see a plane flying at 2000 feet and pick out the logo and its colour painted on the tail!

• Observations from other patients as well as the one above: When the grey 'cloud' dispersed, they had bright flashes of sight in each eye as the nerve fibre was innervated after the opacity drained off and left the eyes a bright natural colour.
• An aperture, or foramina, posteromedial to the caruncle, appears to drain the orbit and lacrimal ducts to the inferior concha of the nasal cavity.
• The suture of the ethmoid bone, medial to the optic nerve, as I massaged the lacrimal gland and tear ducts, the fluid drained obliquely to the pharyngeal, palatine and lingual tonsils to the deep lymphatic chains in the neck. The tear ducts discharged a copious amount of colloidin prior to the watery tears draining into the lymphatics.

- When the drainage occurred, a flow of mucus through the nose and eyes cleared the vessels and glands surrounding the eyeball and lymphatic vessels.
- The above treatment cleared the vessels of the Australian patient to the extent that he could read the medium sized print in a magazine cover about 8–10 feet away without glasses.
- Nerve pain manifests through the increased size of the blocked vessels and diminishes the space required by the optic nerve to transmit the impulses to maintain sight.
- The foreign particulate is lodged in the lymphatic vessels within the back of the orbit, which fibrillates the optic nerve and diminishes the blood supply. Small blood vessels and capillaries rupture to release small amounts of blood into the aqueous humour and the spots and squiggles are formed.

Gangrene (Dry)

Approximately 24 years ago, I was bitten on the right leg by a scorpion. As it apparently healed after a week or so, I did not get medical treatment. Every year or two, I would have problems with recurrent swelling of the affected leg, feeling nauseous and at times, lapsing into an unconscious state. Three years after the attack, I suffered severe hearing loss and the left tarsi drooped over the eye. These attacks would re-occur approximately every two years.

The last attack was in 1996, when lesions the size of a walnut appeared on the affected leg. The first three digits on the foot turned black, and I was in considerable pain. After the lesions healed, the skin on the three affected toes dried and cracked. The bottom pad of the first digit came off in five sections down to the subcutaneous tissue. At that level, there were two medium size lesions. I worked the exudate out and the toe went back to a normal colour.

When I massaged the second and third digits, all the skin on the top of the toes lifted and I had the same result as I did with the first digit. All three eventually went back to their normal colour and had healed within twenty-four hours. There was no necessity for amputation.

I have not had any subsequent problems since the attack described above. The deep lymphatic system is again functioning and fractionizing, liquefying and neutralizing any debris that would cause a blockage, which would prevent the blood from flowing freely.

Gangrene (Wet)

In 1961, my husband carted some heavy strainer posts to a friend's property at Piccadilly in the Adelaide Hills to fix a fence in a horse paddock. As he unloaded the posts and took the weight from the tip truck tray to the ground, he slipped on the wet grass, which sent him off balance as he stopped the posts from sliding down the hill. When he came home, I applied hot foments and massaged on the affected muscles until the pain eased. Apparently, the injury was deep in the perineum because about a week or two later, a boil manifested in the muscles between the testicles and anus.

We called the doctor to our home because he could not sit in a motor vehicle to visit the surgery. After the doctor examined my husband, he wanted him admitted to hospital to put him in a hot bath to relieve the pain. I showed the doctor how we were treating it with massage and steam heat from the foments. The doctor agreed that I should continue with this treatment because of the trauma of transportation to hospital. By treating this at home, I was able to maximize the heat to whatever degree was needed to ease the pain and draw out the exudate which formed the boil. The doctor visited every day to monitor the progress. I applied heat every 2 hours, day and night for the relief of pain.

At the third day, both bowel and bladder ceased to function. To aid urination, pads were placed on the transtubercular plane for about 20 minutes to allow the urine to seep through the sphincter of the bladder as my husband sat on the side of the bed. I would then lightly massage around the boil to push the accumulating debris towards the apex of the boil, but never touch it. Only fluids, boiled bread and milk with plenty of sugar were ingested to maintain strength and minimise the bulk of food ingested. On the seventh day, the doctor lanced the boil, but it was too early. After the incision healed, there appeared to be an excessive amount of scar tissue and nerve pain, which never disappeared.

Twelve months later, another lesion appeared on the scar tissue of the lanced boil. The doctor again visited every day and the same treatment administered. Bowel and bladder function again stopped on the third day. Hot foments were again used to relieve the bladder. On the ninth day the 'lesion' burst, but this time it was a carbuncle. Its 'body' was the size of a walnut with five vessels attached. Approximately half a litre of putrescent pustular secretion, blood and water seeped away from the open wound at the side of the anal sphincter.

Half an hour later, both bowel and bladder functioned. Within three hours of the black putrescent faeces, gel and water passing out of the body, and the return of urination, the cavity tissue had turned black, with streaks of green and yellow gel lesions within. The rectum was visible through the wound.

Apparently, a germ or bacteria had lodged in the wound from the putrescent faeces. I immediately started using the pads again, with their temperature at 212°F and continued work for twelve hours without stopping. As I used the pads, I worked from the healthy tissue back towards the gangrenous centre of the wound. The pain of the gangrenous centre of the lesion was extremely severe and I had to heat the pads to 212°F, which I placed only on the affected area, to try and reduce the level of pain. My contention was: work from the outwards to within to prevent the 'thing', whatever it was, from necrotizing the healthy tissue and applying the pads at 212°F would kill the exudate. My intuition paid off, because after nine hours work, a small pink spot manifested in the centre of the diseased cavity. When the healthy spot appeared, it took another three hours to kill the black, green and yellow substance from the tissue. My husband went back to driving a truck eight days later.

During the time spent treating the above, my husband's legs and body swelled up with the retention of fluid. That too drained to allow the limbs and body to go back to normal size.

At the time of the above trauma, I knew nothing of the lymphatic system, its role in the maintenance of the body, or how it worked or in which direction it flowed. It took another fifteen years of study and practical work to learn the importance of this system, in which direction it drained and the fractionization, liquefaction and the neutralization of the toxic exudate before it re-entered the bloodstream.

Gout

I have written some notes from information held at the Adelaide University, Australia, to help with the information below on how to treat this condition and where.

1. Gutta – in Latin, means a drop from defluxion (a gout-type of pain in big toe).
2. Sudden disappearance (this would occur if the drainage of foreign particulate cleared from the fluid pathways).
3. A copious discharge as of catarrh (which meant if the foreign particulate, which resembled a catarrhal discharge was cleared from the lymphatic pathways).
4. The falling out (as of hair) of the humors. I did not understand the logic of this statement; and I still do not comprehend the meaning!

The term 'podagra' was used if the feet were affected. This is quite simple. If the feet are affected, the first parts to be examined for blockage in the drainage are the feet, legs and perineum.

The inflammation and tophaceous deposits in bone which is a 'sand' or 'grit' in cortical and trabeculated bone structure, proliferates if the bone nutrients, chemicals and minerals pulsation into the interstitium is restricted by the blocked drainage. The bone 'dies' and degrades to a sequestrum.

It is the joints, rather than the bones, which are the sites of major lesions in gout in the locomotor system. The deposition of urates, the diamine of carbonic acid found in urine, blood and lymph and the chief nitrogenous end product of protein metabolis is formed in the liver from amino acids and ammonia compounds that causes an inflammatory and cell reaction in tissues and bone. It creates an acidic burning, vibratory pain similar to arthritis if the above exudate circulates around the nerve fibres.

When the manifestation of the above occurs, the first system I suspect of dysfunction is the lymphatic plexuses, vessels and nodes surrounding the digestive system in the cheeks, throat, tongue, oesophagus, stomach, duodenum, jejunum, spleen, pancreas and liver. If any of the glands in and around any of the above organs dysfunction, the enzymes, digastric juices and hormonal secretions imbalance from the lymphatic blockage, malfunction to the extent that metabolism, anabolism and catabolism, the breaking down of molecules of nutrients to be absorbed into the blood, is inhibited. This provokes the inflammatory and cellular reaction from what I see as being from the excessive amounts of acid in the interstitial fluid.

Medical research has not proved that an attack of gout is occasioned by a new deposition of urates in the tissues. Chronic manifestations are dependent on this phenomenon. However, if the natural killer and filtration cells in the lymph nodes are dysfunctioning from the drainage of fluids being inhibited, failure to fractionize, liquefy and neutralize any of the particulate causing the problem, it would lead to a continual build-up and maintain an excessively high level of acidity.

Gout is characterised by articular inflammation from microcrystals of monosodium urate monohydrate in the joints, and the deposits of tophi, a chalky deposit in joints and kidneys.

Hyperuricemia, an excess of uric acid in the blood, is determined by the rates of production and elimination of urate. Purine, a heterocyclic compound in homo sapiens, produces uric acid. Microcrystals of monosodium urate monohydrate in joints and deposits of chalky deposit in joints and kidneys. Microcrystals resemble salt or sugar grains immersed in plasma an amber coloured oil substance produced in the diaphysis of bone. Insoluble at body temperature (98.4°F) but will liquefy with the application of hot foments from 130–180°F and drain.

If the body systems are dysfunctioning, micro-crystals as in dystrophic calcification, form in the membrane-bound cells derived from degenerating cells, will be deposited in the joints with the bacteria, dead bone cells and bone marrow debris, as it does in arthritis.

As I treat patients with gout, arthritis, osteoporosis, and other inflammatory 'diseases', I note the following for gout. The colour of the toes, the size and look of the ankle joint and sometimes a fluid retention in the leg from the toes to the inguinals and the articular joints will have a reddish brown translucent appearance. I lightly massage the whole leg from the feet upward with a flat-hand action – this is less painful than any other manipulation. I use steam heat on the swelling, which gives quick relief. If the fluid is retained in the cellular tissues, it degenerates and gels.

As it is highly acidic, the action of the acids and the pressure of excess fluids, fibrillates the nerve impulses from the brain to the motor end plates of the fibres and causes a burning, stinging, vibratory pain in the surrounding musculature.

As work progresses on the superficial, medial and deep lymphatics in the direction of the flow, the fifteen natural killer cells of the lymph nodes will purify the fluid before it re-enters the bloodstream, after passing through 8–10 lymph nodes for purification.

Dystrophic calcification can be intracellular and extracellular, and can progress to bone formations. I have noted the transformation of calcification into bone while treating patients with arthritis. It is also evident in X-rays as the particulate shows a white image, completely obliterating the shape of any part of the skeleton and cellular tissue.

Hydroxyapitite crystals, an inorganic constituent matrix of bone, and the calcified tissue cells form a plaque between the bones. The tophi, being a gritty substance, combined with the hydroxyapatite crystals, wears both the synovial and cartilage down to the opposing bone surfaces that fuse together. Collagen, the main component in cartilage, also enhances crystal production and acts as a sign of an earlier injury, especially in osteoporosis.

Gout is easier to treat than arthritis, as it does not calcify. To treat a gouty patient, practitioners must be aware of the direction of flow in the interstitium before it is propelled into the deep lymphatic vessels.

Full body treatment must be given. The quantity of urine increases and an acidic reaction may be noticed by the patient. Nerve pain may also present as the acidic particulate is drained from around the nerve fibres, as massage, with steam heat, progresses. I use extra hot foments to liquefy the gel and bring relief more quickly.

Usually, after the fourth treatment, the reduction in quantity of fluid relieves the pressure on the nerves. The length of time to effect a cure is relative to the chronicity of the complaint. Some patients will only take about three months and others will take twelve months. Full body massage must be given to clear all fluid outlets to activate the kidneys and other organs.

Hodgkin's Disease

Hodgkin's disease is so-called after Thomas Hodgkin (1798–1866) the Guy's Hospital pathologist who first described it as lymphandenoma. Hodgkin's Disease is a chronic disorder caused by the enlargement of lymph nodes at the base of the occipital, root of the neck, axillary nodes and inguinals. The cause of the complaint is not well-known medically.

The lymphatic chains from the base of the skull form the deep plexuses along the cervicals to the root of the neck. It has been treated successfully, working on the deep vessels, by specialized massage and steam heat from hot foments, heated in a microwave oven or a machine with a wringer attached. Massage and steam heat is initiated from the occipital bone, atlas and axis, through the cranial and cervicals and muscular tissue down to the root of the neck, clavicle, scapulae and the first two ribs.

The 'disease' has been found predominantly in patients who have had an accident or traumatic birth by the doctor using forceps to deliver the baby. Again, as in other conditions, the muscle and ligament fibres are pulled out of the root canals in the bone and the tissue cells are ruptured.

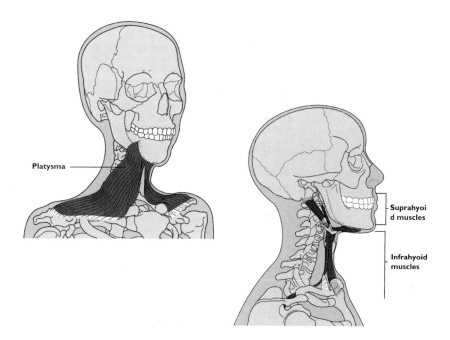

Platysma

Suprahyoid muscles

Infrahyoid muscles

Figure 54: Some of the head, throat, neck and shoulder muscles affected by Hodgkin's disease.

Bone protein, plasma and water, minerals, chemicals and nutrients calcify when penetrated by the calcium from the tissues and phosphates stored in the mitochondria of ruptured cells. The exudate will form an ectopic or dystrophic calcification, which fibrillates the nerve impulse sent from the brain to the motor end plates within the muscles. It shows a white shadow in X-rays and scans.

I have also noted an amyloid protein – a fatty, waxy, starchy substance – formed within the brain, covering the periosteal surface of the bone. This prevents nutrients, chemicals and minerals, transported in the interstitial fluid, entering the nutrient canals of the skeletal structure. It also inhibits circulation of fluids in the cellular environment.

As I work on the deep lymphatic vessels affected by Hodgkin's disease, I find the plexuses at the base of the skull and the foramina in the bony labyrinth are blocked by the amyloid protein and ectopic calcification. All the cranial nerves are fibrillated, which causes loss of balance, sight disturbance, speech defects, headaches, deglutition of solids and liquids because of little or no innervation to activate the muscles of control.

I work in the direction of the deep lymphatic flow before and after the application of steam heated pads to drain the liquefied 'insoluble' foreign particulate away from the affected areas. The patient will have slight trauma as the coagulated foreign particulate is massaged through the microscopic tubules and nodes in the plexuses.

The deep lymphatic vessels that drain the meninges also traverse through the foramina, into the deep lymphatic chains on the cranial and cervical bones. The deep lymphatics from the brain that drain into the cerebral vessels, through the foramen magnum, also empty into the deep lymphatics on the cranial and cervical bones.

As work progresses with the heat and massage, the interstitial fluid pulsates into the interstitium by the systolic pressure of the cardiac cycle, and is absorbed into the semi-liquefied foreign particulate, which facilitates its removal before it necrotizes and eliminates any possibility of malignant cells forming.

Steam heat is essential when massaging the fibrillated nerves of the cranium because, with manipulation alone, there could be an adverse reaction when the small vessels become overloaded without liquefaction. I find the steam heat is more effective and with less patient trauma, when the coagulant, either blood, foreign particulate or gelled interstitial fluid liquefies and drains into the blind-ending valved ducts. I also find it essential to give full body treatment, as I have noticed in all upper region problems, that the foreign debris will drain into plexuses in the lower part of the body and set up adverse reactions elsewhere, if only the affected parts are massaged (**see** also Parkinson's disease).

Kidney Stones

I treated a patient approximately twenty years ago, who had severe pain across thoracic 9–12 and lumbar 1–5 around the kidneys and the right lobe of liver. He informed me that he has had recurrent bouts of severe pain for twenty-six years and had been hospitalised once although nothing definite had been diagnosed.

To treat the patient, he laid prone on the plinth. I gave a full treatment from feet to head but did not find the cause of the pain. I then requested he lay on his side. I immediately found the basic cause of the problem. I worked on the obliquus muscles that were attached to the ribcage, spine and iliac crest over the kidneys and had a positive response on both the left and right muscles.

I then requested he lay supine for further examination. The pain was acute over omentum and under rectus abdominis at the site of the lymphatic plexuses both lateral and level with the umbilicus. I applied a lot of steam heated foments interspersed with gentle flat-hand massage. I continued this treatment for three hours which produced a slight relief from pain. I requested that his wife repeat the treatment for about an hour before retiring to bed.

He came back the next morning and I repeated the above work for three hours. I sent him home for a short rest before his wife gave a short treatment in the afternoon and again at night before retiring to bed.

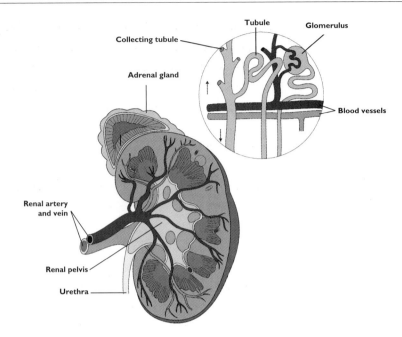

Figure 55: A cross-section of the kidney.

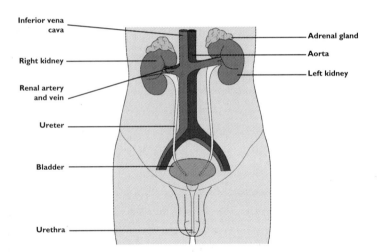

Figure 56: The urinary system.

On the third day he came in the morning, and I gave him a short treatment of about one hour and sent him home. At this stage he had a lot of relief from pain. As I worked on the side over the obliquus muscles, an obstruction which felt very hard and about the size of a broad bean seed moved from where it was embedded in or near the hilum of the ureter.

The next morning while having a shower he felt a hard, immovable obstruction in or near the sphincter of the urethra and penis. He manipulated it through the penis and the kidney stone fell onto the floor of the shower recess. The stone was the shape of the ureter at the fluid exit of the kidney. It was 20mms long and 12mms wide. The patient has not had any more trouble for twenty years.

Lower Back Pain

When a patient presents with a paralyzing pain from the ischium/ilium, up to lumbar 1, and in the oblique muscles between the ribcage and ilium, I observe their movements when they try to walk or sit. The sharp 'nerve' pain in the vertebrae inhibits free movement.

Pain is initiated by three systems – the nervous system, the muscle roots at both insertions and origins into the bone, and the dysfunctioning lymphatic system.

If possible, lie the patient on a plinth – prone, supine or on their side – the site of the pain is at the location of the following muscles, ligaments and tendons:

1.   Quadratus lumborum – its origins at the posterior part of the crest of the ilium and inserts into the lower ribs.

2.   Iliocostalis muscles – lateral division of erector muscle of spine and angles of lower 6 ribs.

3.   Iliocostalis lumborum – a thick tendon. The origins are from the sacrum, T11 and T12 vertebrae, the spinous processes of the lumbar and the medial lips of the iliac crest. Its insertions are at the inferior borders of the angles of the lower 6th and 7th ribs.

4.   Longissimus thoracis – a common thick tendon with the iliocostalis lumborum, fibres from the transverse and accessory processes of the lumbar vertebrae and the lumbodorsal fascia.

5.   Serratus posterior inferior – origins are spinous processes of T11, T12 and L1, 2 and 3 of the lumbodorsal fascia. The insertions are on the inferior borders of the lower 4 ribs, just beyond their angles.

6.   Transversus abdominis – the origin is the lateral half of the inguinal ligament, anterior ⅔ of inner lips of the iliac crest, lumbodorsal fascia and from the inner edges of the lower 6 costal cartilages. The insertions are at the linea alba and its aponeurosis. I have marked two lymphatic plexuses - both lateral to the linea alba and umbilicus.

7.   Rectus abdominis – the origin is at the pubic crest and symphysis pubis. The insertions are at ribs 5, 6 and 7 and at the side of the xiphoid process. The lymphatic plexuses marked on the transversus abdominis lie posterior to the rectus abdominis and the downward drainage from the parasternals drain into the marked plexuses.

8.   Internal lateral oblique (anterior division) – the origins at the lateral ⅔ of the inguinal ligament and the anterior ⅓ of the middle (or intermediate line) of the iliac crest. The insertions are at the crest of the pubis and the linea alba and its aponeurosis.

9.   The internal obliquus (abdominal) lateral division – the origin is the middle ⅓ of the iliac crest on the mid-line and the lumbodorsal fascia. The insertion is at the inferior borders of the 10th, 11th and 12th ribs.

10. External abdominal oblique – he origins are the external surfaces and inferior borders of ribs 5–12 by tendinous slips that interdigitate with those of serratus anterior and latissimus dorsi. Insertions are at linea alba by means of the broad aponeurosis from the ribs to the crest of the pubis, inguinal ligament and the anterior half of the iliac crest, along the outer lip.

11. Sheath of rectus abdominis – the aponeurosis of the transversus abdominis, internal oblique and external oblique.

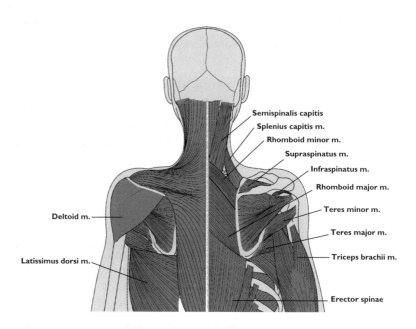

Figure 57: Muscles of the back.

The direction in which the lymphatic system drains is important to enable practitioners to either treat lower back pain and effect a cure or just give relief from pain. Other parts of the body, whether homo sapiens or quadrupeds, will respond to DLT if worked in the direction of the flow. Blood, lymph and nerves lie in close proximity to each other in all parts of the body.

It will be noted that there are different levels of flow to drain the wastes of metabolism, anabolism and catabolism of nutrients, chemicals, minerals, dead cells and any bacteria that enter the body, which, depending upon the exudate and presence of inhibiting factors, will be excreted through the bowel and bladder.

Pain is exacerbated in all parts of the anatomy if the patient has had an accident, is traumatized by playing sport to the extent muscles and ligaments are injured, or develops pain and stress from postural fatigue whilst sitting in chairs not designed for their specific job. The muscles and ligament fibres and their origins and insertions into bone will either pull away from the root canals in the bone or rupture. The nerve impulses from the brain to the individual fibres will be fibrillated through the accident or by the accumulated foreign debris at the site of the injury.

As I treat a lower back pain patient, I note their reactions. I work on the musculature from the knee upwards, through the gluteals and obliquus muscles to the ribcage because the bone where the muscles and ligaments attach and have been pulled out or ruptured is very painful. My questions were:

1.   What is the obstruction?
2.   What and why is it always at the muscle attachments?
3.   What is the foreign particulate that always accumulates on the bone?
4.   Why any type of accident, whether they fell on a hard surface, twisting the pelvic bones at the transtubercular plane, or twisting the spine at the transpyloric plane?

The amyloid protein 'seeps' through the canals in the bones from the occipital to the coccyx out of the arachnoid space between pia mater of the medulla and the dura mater of the vertebrae. An ectopic or dystrophic calcification can be seen in the muscles, which have either been stretched or ruptured from the canals in the bone surface, and will be seen as a white shadow in the extracellular tissue, as seen in X-rays and scans. As the damaged cell necrotizes from the injury, calcium from the tissues enters the degenerated cells and combines with the phosphates stored

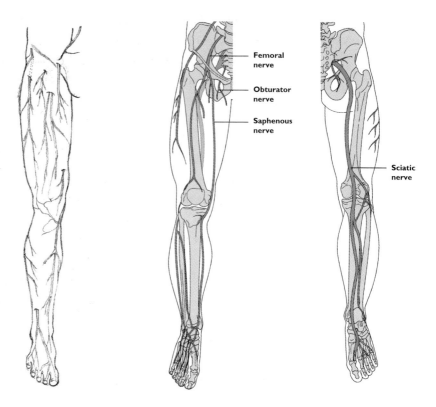

Figure 58: Nerves affected by lymphatic blockage in inguinals and trochanter. Vessels lie transversely from the base of trochanter. One vessel drains into perineum at adductor magnus muscle; the second drainage enters 2 inguinal nodes anterior of thigh. The blocked drainage fibrillates the femoral, saphenous, obturator and the twigs and branches from these nerves partially fibrillate the sciatic nerve.

in the mitochondria to form hydroxyapatite crystals. This is also enhanced by the addition of the gelled collagen as the cells are ruptured. The coagulant from the injured blood vessels also create a blockage that prevents the interstitial fluid from draining into the interstitium from the fenestrated muscles of the veins and capillaries.

An aerobe, a micro-organism formed in the injured cells, will absorb the oxygen in the surrounding tissue cells. The denuded cells then form an anaerobic enzyme which fractionizes and liquefies the dead cells, which has been denuded of oxygen at the site of the injury. The deep lymphatics dysfunction and the decomposed acidic foreign particulate remain within the striations of the muscles fibres. The fibrillation of the impulse from the above injury causes an acidic stinging, burning, vibratory pain that is associated with lower back pain and other arthritic 'diseases'.

Treatment

To treat a lower back pain patient, he/she should lie prone on the plinth or on their side if the prone position is too painful. Hot foments are used with specific massage on the hips, obliquus muscles and ribcage at the origins and insertions of the muscles and ligaments listed. I also massage the deep lymphatic vessels that drain downwards from the occipital to the coccyx, between the spinous process and the transverse spines. A collagenous exudate and what feels like amyloid (a fatty, waxy, starchy protein, found in plaques in the brain and other organs) covers the nutrient canals in the vertebrae as it seeps from the arachnoid spaces and covers the bone surfaces. The main concentrations of amyloid are from:

1. The occipital over the cranial, cervical and down to the 8th thoracic which I noted when treating osteoporosis patients.
2. About the 2nd lumbar, down to the 3rd sacrum in lower back pain patients. It flows laterally left and right, over the iliac crest, where lesions from the size a pea to a broad bean form, and are attached to the bone by vessels. As these obstructions 'grow', they fibrillate the lumbar/sacral plexuses.

The foreign particulate is difficult to treat and surgery does not appear to be a success, because all the patients I have treated after surgical intervention have continual pain after the operation.

Some patients respond to this treatment immediately whilst others take longer. Although pain is relieved at the first treatment, the treatment takes from three to six months. If the patients' condition is chronic, I treat twice a week, two hourly sessions for four treatments, and then revert back to once a week. No operations are necessary.

Other conditions causing back pain are when a fall, kick or a twist of muscles has injured the gluteals. The same phenomenon occurs when the muscle attachments have been ruptured or torn from the bone.

There are two deep lymphatic vessels between the gluteus maximus, medius and minimus. The vessels lie on the periosteum, from the sacrum, and drain laterally to a plexus surrounding the trochanter, neck of femur and iliac crest. Gluteus minimus has a separate drainage vessel that runs parallel to the other gluteal vessel into the same plexus. The foreign particulate is then drained by other vessels into the inguinal nodes and glands, where it is drained through the perineum into the glands below the cysterna chyli and thoracic duct.

There is also a deep lymphatic drainage between the spinous process and transverse spines. Its origins begin at the deep cervical chains from the bony labyrinth of the occipital, atlas and axis bones on the left and right sides, down to the coccygeal plexus. The left and right drainage vessels are joined together below the coccyx and the combined drainage flows back towards the lymph glands before entering the cysterna chyli and thoracic duct. If an excess of drainage is evident, the patient will have pain as the fluid traverses in close proximity to the obturator nerve, piriformis muscle and obturator foramen, down through the adductor magnus muscles, to the medial side of the knee joint. The flow of interstitial fluid and lymph in the obliquus muscles will slow down and gel. The fibrillation, as in all other parts of the body, causes a stinging, burning, vibratory pain from the coccyx up to the sacrum and lumbar. The intensity of pain registers at the dorsal roots' entrance to the medulla. In every patient, I find the source of pain is from the blocked drainage in quadratus lumborum whose origins are from the iliac crest and the lumbodorsal fascia. Its insertions are at the 12th rib and transverse processes of the lumbar vertebrae. Its innervations arise from the 12th thoracic, 1st and 2nd lumbar. The blocked muscle fibres are very prominent and can be easily massaged transversely, both supine and prone. The patient immediately has pain where the dorsal nerve roots enter the medulla. Steam heat and massage removes the problem that fibrillates the nerves. The muscles are activated to propel the foreign particulate that is causing the fibrillation into the blind-ending valved ducts of the deep lymphatic vessels.

The nerves most affected by the calcification and amyloid protein seepage are the iliohypogastric, iliolingual, genito-femoral, lateral cutaneous of thigh obturator, lumbo-sacral trunk, femoral and saphenous. They are all, including the sciatic nerve roots, connected by twigs and branches. The lateral cutaneous and femoral nerves appear to give the most pain down the leg laterally to the 5th digit on the foot. Medially, the obturator acts with the synergists, piriformis, obturator externus and internus and the superior and inferior gemelli. The pain of the fibrillated obturator goes from its origins in the roots of the lumbar plexus from L1, down through the sciatic roots, and then traverses deep through the obturator foramen and extends to the medial side of the knee joint.

The sacral plexus is formed by the anterior rami, the three sacral nerve roots and the 4th and 5th lumbar roots from which the sciatic nerve arises. The fine lymphatic plexuses serve every layer of skin in which there are the following layers:

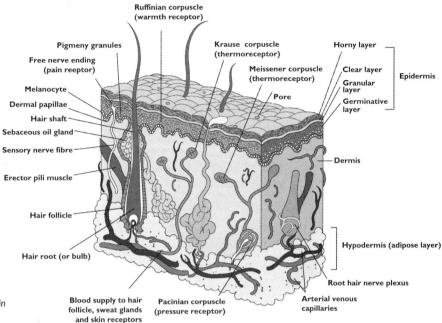

Ruffinian corpuscle
(warmth receptor)

Pigmeny granules

Free nerve ending
(pain reeptor)

Melanocyte

Dermal papillae

Hair shaft

Sebaceous oil gland

Sensory nerve fibre

Erector pili muscle

Hair follicle

Hair root (or bulb)

Krause corpuscle
(thermoreceptor)

Meissener corpuscle
(thermoreceptor)

Pore

Horny layer

Clear layer

Granular
layer

Germinative
layer

Epidermis

Dermis

Hypodermis (adipose layer)

Root hair nerve plexus

Blood supply to hair
follicle, sweat glands
and skin receptors

Pacinian corpuscle
(pressure receptor)

Arterial venous
capillaries

Figure 59: Diagram of the skin and subcutaneous tissue.

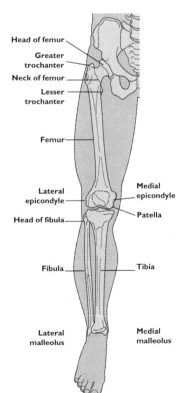

Head of femur

Greater
trochanter

Neck of femur

Lesser
trochanter

Femur

Lateral
epicondyle

Head of fibula

Fibula

Lateral
malleolus

Medial
epicondyle

Patella

Tibia

Medial
malleolus

Figure 60: Bones of the leg and hip.

1. Stratum corneum;

2. Stratum lucidum;

3. Stratum granulosum;

4. Stratum spinosum;

5. Stratum germinativum.

I find the fine lymphatics serve every layer of skin as Professor Neil Piller, Flinders University, Adelaide demonstrated on videos and slides at a seminar. The cardiac cycle pulsation and peristaltic action of the diaphragm propels the foreign debris into the valves of the blind ending ducts which relieves the pressure of toxins on the nerves in the musculature.

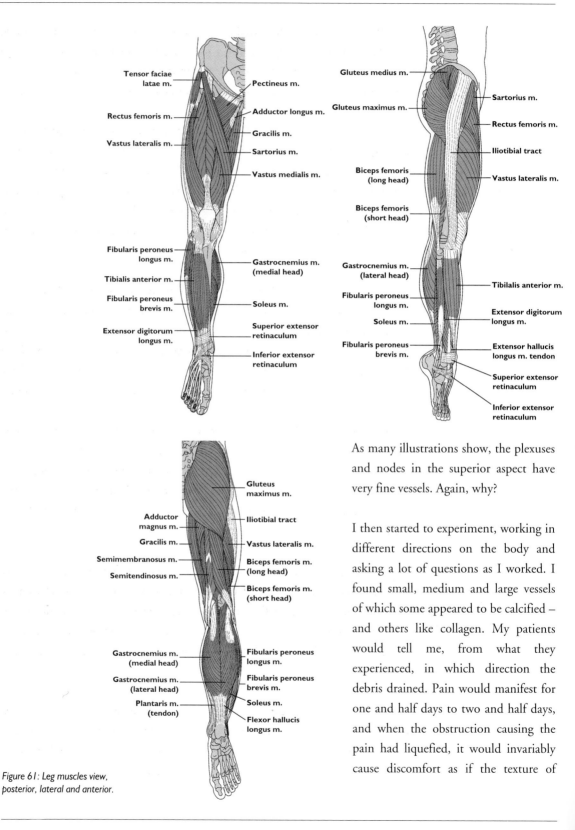

Tensor faciae latae m.
Pectineus m.
Rectus femoris m.
Adductor longus m.
Vastus lateralis m.
Gracilis m.
Sartorius m.
Vastus medialis m.
Fibularis peroneus longus m.
Tibialis anterior m.
Gastrocnemius m. (medial head)
Fibularis peroneus brevis m.
Soleus m.
Extensor digitorum longus m.
Superior extensor retinaculum
Inferior extensor retinaculum

Gluteus medius m.
Gluteus maximus m.
Sartorius m.
Rectus femoris m.
Iliotibial tract
Biceps femoris (long head)
Vastus lateralis m.
Biceps femoris (short head)
Gastrocnemius m. (lateral head)
Fibularis peroneus longus m.
Tibialis anterior m.
Soleus m.
Extensor digitorum longus m.
Fibularis peroneus brevis m.
Extensor hallucis longus m. tendon
Superior extensor retinaculum
Inferior extensor retinaculum

Gluteus maximus m.
Adductor magnus m.
Iliotibial tract
Gracilis m.
Vastus lateralis m.
Semimembranosus m.
Biceps femoris m. (long head)
Semitendinosus m.
Biceps femoris m. (short head)
Gastrocnemius m. (medial head)
Fibularis peroneus longus m.
Gastrocnemius m. (lateral head)
Fibularis peroneus brevis m.
Plantaris m. (tendon)
Soleus m.
Flexor hallucis longus m.

Figure 61: Leg muscles view, posterior, lateral and anterior.

As many illustrations show, the plexuses and nodes in the superior aspect have very fine vessels. Again, why?

I then started to experiment, working in different directions on the body and asking a lot of questions as I worked. I found small, medium and large vessels of which some appeared to be calcified – and others like collagen. My patients would tell me, from what they experienced, in which direction the debris drained. Pain would manifest for one and half days to two and half days, and when the obstruction causing the pain had liquefied, it would invariably cause discomfort as if the texture of whatever it was, was too thick to drain through a vessel that was so small. Finally, the blockage would be propelled into a much larger vessel by the liquefied foreign particulate and the additional normal interstitial fluid pulsated into the interstitium. The pain would subside as the blockage dissipated.

It took thirty-five years to find the answers to all of my questions and I am still learning! On each side of the umbilicus, in the obliquus muscles, a lymph plexus, as noted by practitioner and patient to be between rectus abdominis and the omentum, forms part of the deep lymphatic chain draining the obliquus muscles and the downward drainage from the parasternals. If the flow through these plexuses is blocked, the motor end plates of the nerves from the lower thoracics, lumbar and upper sacrum fibrillates which is part of low back pain.

The treatment of the obliquus muscles described above, together with the treatment of the legs is essential to relieve lower back pain. Both left and right legs have to be treated equally. The patient will lie on their side on a plinth, curve the leg to be treated, which is placed on a cushion to elevate the knee and relieve the tension of the muscles. I place both hands together to use the pads of the thumbs on the leg with fingers stabilizing the pressure each side to alleviate pain.

I stand at the foot of the plinth and work from the lateral malleoleus with thumbs between the muscles up to the knee joint. I then go to the side of the plinth and place my thumbs on the origins of the iliotibial tract in tibia. I work between the individual muscles of the leg and directly over the iliotibial tract, trochanter, tensor fascia latae and the gluteals to the iliac spine and crest, both posterolateral and anterolateral.

When working as above, both practitioners and patient will observe at the origins of the iliotibial tract a plaque of detritus. This consists of a tough collagenous powdery chalk particulate; a third to half way up the femur, calcified nodules, like grains of wheat on the bone and at the roots of the muscles; and, at the base of the trochanter, large calcified vessels lying transversely, draining towards the inguinal glands.

Above the trochanter, calcified vessels arising from the tensor fascia latae and iliac crest drain medially to the abdominal cavity at the transtubercular plane into the inguinal glands. The vessels and glands, when 'overloaded' from the downward drainage from the rectus abdominis, omentum and iliac crest, will cause sharp

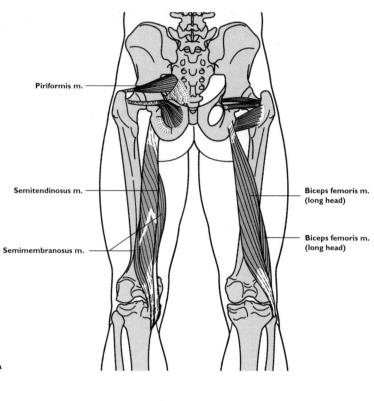

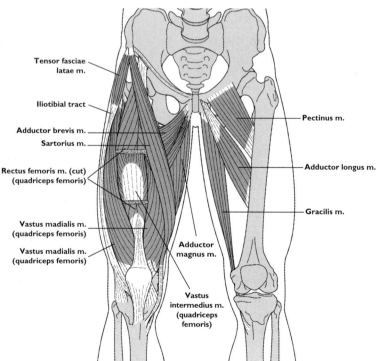

Figure 62: Deep muscles of the leg anterior, posterior.

stabbing pains in the groin when the patient tries to stand erect. Practitioners will, after working anterially, go to the posterior and work from the iliac crest over the trochanter down to below the knee joint.

The use of steam heated foments is essential between massages to liquefy the fragmented foreign particles in the detritus as the work progresses, and drainage will be facilitated and processed by the lymphatic apparatus. Massage and the use of steam heated foments as described on the obliquus muscles and legs will render the use of drugs and operations unnecessary. Here are some origins and insertions into bone that may be of assistance to the practitioner.

Muscles

Sartorius	Innervation – L2, L3; origin – anterior superior spine of iliac crest; insertion – medial surface of body of tibia.
Gracilis	Innervation – L2, L3; origin – anterior of lower half of symphysis pubis; insertion – medial surface of body of tibia.
Biceps Femoris	Innervation – lateral hamstring L5, S1, S2; origin – long head from ischial tuberosity, short head – sacrotuberous ligament; insertion – head of fibula and lateral condyle of tibia.
Semitendinosus	Innervation – tibial nerve from sciatic nerve; origin – ischial tuberosity with tendon of long head of biceps femoris; insertion – anterior and medial surface of tibia below condyle.
Semimembranosus	Innervation – tibial nerve from sciatic nerve; origin – upper and lateral aspect of ischial tuberosity; insertion – posterior surface of medial condyle of tibia.
Rectus Femoris	Innervation – femoral nerve; origin – anterior inferior iliac spine; insertion – upper border or patella.

Vastus Lateralis

Innervation – femoral nerve; origin – head of femur; insertion – tibial tuberosity through patellar ligament.

Popliteus

Innervation – tibial nerve; origin – lateral condyle of femur; insertion – patella, posterior surface of tibia.

Extensor Digitorum

Longus Innervation – deep peroneal nerve; origin – lateral condyle of tibia head and proximal of anterior surface on fibula and interosseous membrane; insertion – divides into four tendons attached to dorsal surfaces of 2nd–5th toes.

Muscle of the Legs

Gluteals

Maximus

Origin – posterior gluteal line of ilium aponeurosis of erector spinae, dorsal surface of sacrum coccyx; sacrotuberous ligament.; insertion – gluteal turberosity of femur and iliotibial tract of tensor fascia latae; nerve supply – L5, S1,2.

Medius

Origin – outer surface of ilium, from iliac crest and posterior gluteal line above to the anterior gluteal line, gluteal aponeurosis; insertion – gluteal tuberosity of femur and iliotibial tract of tensor fascia latae; nerve supply – L5, S1.

Minimus

Origin – outer surface of ilium between anterior and inferior gluteal line and the margin of the greater sciatic notch; insertion – anterior border of the greater trochanter; nerve supply – L5, S1.

Tensor Fascia Latae

Origin – anterior part of the outer lip of the iliac crest, outer surface of anterior superior iliac spine; insertion – iliotibial band of fascia latae on the anteriolateral aspect of the thigh, about a third of the way down; nerve supply – L4, 5, S1.

Tibialis Posterior	Origin – lateral part of posterior surface of the tibia proximal, two thirds of medial surface of fibula; insertion – tuberosity of navicular with branches to calcaneus, cuneiforms and cuboid and bases of 2nd, 3rd and 4th metatarsals; nerve supply – L5, S1, 2.
Peroneus Longus	Origin – head and proximal two-thirds of lateral surface of fibula intermuscular septa and adjacent fascia; insertion – lateral margin of plantar surface of 1st cuneiform and base of 1st metatarsal; nerve supply – L5, S1, 2.
Peroneus Tertius	Origin – distal 3rd of the anterior surface of the fibula; insertion – dorsal surface of the 5th metatarsal; nerve supply – L5, S1.
Peroneus Brevis	Origin – distal two-thirds of lateral surface of the body of fibula and septa; insertion – tuberosity on the lateral side base of the 5th metatarsal; nerve supply – L5, S1.
Gastrocnemius	Origin – lateral condyle and posterior surface of the femur; capsule of the knee joint; insertion – posterior surface of calcaneus by Achilles tendon; nerve supply – tibial, S1, 2.
Psoas Major	Origin – anterior surface of the transverse process, lateral borders of vertebral bodies and intervertebral discs of T12, L5; insertion – lesser trochanter of femur and along medial border of shaft; nerve supply – lumbar plexus, L1, 2, 3.
Iliacus	Origin – superior two-thirds of iliac fossa, inner lip of iliac crest, anterior sacroiliac, lumbosacral, iliolumbar ligaments, all of sacrum; insertion – lesser trochanter of the femur and below, along medial border of shaft; nerve supply – femoral, L2, 3.

Vastus Medialis	Origin – lower half of the trochanteric line, medial lip of linea aspera, upper part of supracondylar line, medial intermuscular septum, tendons of adductor magnus and longus; insertion – medial border of patella, through the ligamentum patellae into tibial tuberosity; nerve supply – femoral, L2, 3, 4.
Vastus Intermedius	Origin – proximal two-thirds of the anterolateral surface of the femur, lower half of linea aspera, upper part of lateral supracondylar line, lateral intermuscular septum; insertion – by tendons of the rectus and vasti muscles into the superior border of the patellar ligament into tibial tuberosity; nerve supply – femoral, L2, 3, 4.
Adductor Brevis	Origin – outer surface of body, inferior ramus of pubis; insertion – extending from the lesser trochanter to the upper line of the linea aspera; nerve supply – obturator, L2, 3, 4.
Adductor Longus	Origin – front of the pubis in the angle between the crest and symphysis pubis; insertion – middle third of the medial lip of linea aspera; nerve supply – obturator, L2, 3, 4.
Adductor Magnus	Origin – *posterior fibres*: ischial tuberosity; *anterior fibres*: ramus of ischium and pubis; insertion – from line extending from the gluteal tuberosity along the linea aspera, medial supracondylar line, adductor tubercle on medial condyle of femur; nerve supply – posterior fibres: tibial portion of sciatic L4, 5, S1; *anterior fibres*: obturator, L2, 3, 4.
Obturator Internis	Origin – pelvic surface of obturator membrane and bony margin of obturator foramen; insertion – medial surface of the greater trochanter; nerve supply – sacral plexus, L5, S1, 2.

Case Study – Fred

A few years ago, a colleague went to the local hotel and whilst he was there, he observed the hotel-keeper grasping the bar and nearly fainting from the extreme pain in his back. A colleague assisted him by performing light massage. He could not relieve the spasm enough to inhibit the pain, as the problem was too deep. The hotel-keeper was also a race horse trainer. I examined him the next day and gave him light treatment with steam heat.

His pain initiated at L3–5 and S1–4. High aggregations of large collagenous obstructions were fibrillating the peripheral nerves from L3 to the coccygeal plexus. A mosaic pattern of blocked lymphatic vessels was also noted on the ribcage; obliquus muscles; gluteus maximus, medius and minimus; downwards from iliac crest anterior/posterior trochanter to the knee joint.

The treatment was given on a weekly basis and relief from pain was noted. I gave full body treatment. The liquefied foreign particulate, if only worked in a small area, would not have any outlet because it could not penetrate the blocked vessels of the deep lymphatics that surround it. I gave him the lower back pain treatment and had freedom from pain at three months and freedom from the problem at six months. I gave treatment for another five months on a fortnightly basis to make sure the deep lymphatics were working normally.

Migraine

A migraine headache is basically the result of an injury causing 'whiplash' by a hard or violent movement such as a car accident, a fall, or birth procedures where forceps have been used when the baby's head has been locked in the birth canal (by cramp of the mother's muscles in Bandl's ring, also referred to as the pathologic retraction ring). This is a complication of a prolonged labour marked by the failure of relaxation of the circular fibres at the internal opening of the cervix, preventing the birth of the infant. By using the forceps, the baby's muscles and ligaments of the head, neck and shoulders have been stretched beyond their capacity. Bone damage also occurs in the skull and cervicals whereby the roots of the transverse ligament will either rupture or tear from the root canals in the bone.

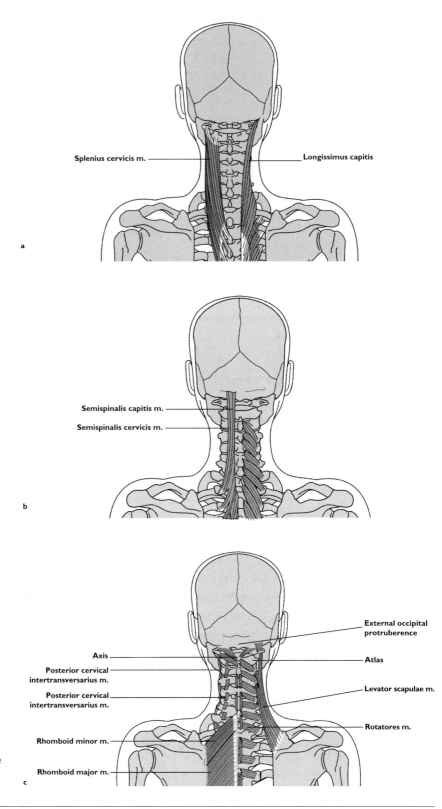

Figure 63: The neck and head muscles affected by blocked lymph drainage causing migraine headaches.

When I treat migraine, I find the main muscles affected by the injury are:

1.   Semispinalis capitis. Origins: Transverse process of the upper thoracic and lower cervicals. Insertion: Temporal bone.
2.   Splenius capitis. Origin: Ligamentum nuchae. Insertion: Temporal bone.
3.   Longissimus capitis. Origins: Transverse processes of the upper thoracic and lower cervicals. Insertion: Temporal bone.

The foreign particulate formed from the leakage of bone protein, dead bone cells and the debris of dead cellular tissue will form an obstruction combined with the gelled plasma in the interstitial fluid. It consolidates into a hard, collagenous, powdery sand plaque.

The plaque surrounds the cranial nerves and fibrillates the nerve impulse from the brain as the fibres transmit the impulse through the foramina lateral to the foramen magnum and into the bony labyrinth of the occipital to innervate the organs connected to the cranial nerves.

This plaque is also responsible for the fibrillation of the nerve blockage in the central nervous system and peripheral nerves that cause the 'flitting skin syndrome', 'violent nocturnal spasms', 'wriggling diaphragm' and 'persistent unexplained nausea'. Treatment for these conditions consists of specialized lymphatic massage in the pathways of the blood and fluid flows, accompanied by the application of dampened woollen blankets, which are heated to a high temperature in a microwave and placed on the patient.

The steam-heated pads liquefy the gelled interstitial fluid and plasma. The interstitial fluid pulsated into the interstitium at 72–80 beats a minute by the cardiac cycle, the vacuum of the airless environment in the blood vascular and deep lymphatic systems all assist the lymphatic massage to propel the liquefied foreign particulate into the blind-ending valved ducts of the lymphatic system. Here, it is fractionized, liquefied and neutralized and then drained into the thoracic duct as pure water.

Case Study – Trixibelle

Several years ago another patient was introduced to me by my colleague. The patient was female, aged forty-eight years old, one of twins and suffered from migraine headaches. She was overweight, had congenital deformities and was in constant pain. She was married and had four children.

Her early history was that her mother had a difficult pregnancy at the birth of the twins. The first twin had both normal growth and presentation. The second twin (patient) oblique (back) presentation; also abnormal foetal position in utero. Her arms appeared to have been pushed above her head and face pushed up and backwards in the placenta to rest on the uterine wall. Ribcage underdeveloped and

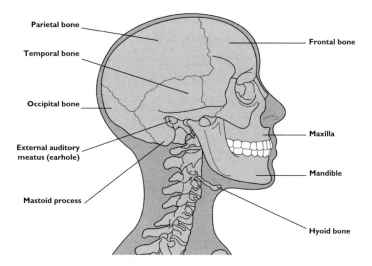

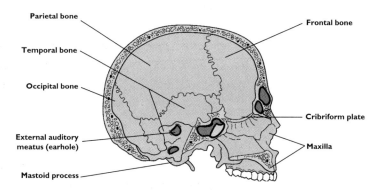

Figure 64: Head and neck bones affected by blocked lymphatic drainage causing migraine headaches.

right humerus 8cms shorter than the left. Cervical transverse spines short and bowed. She was a difficult baby to rear, constantly crying, feeding problems and overweight. She suffered health problems to adulthood.

When pregnant with her first baby, many problems presented. The baby went full term but was stillborn at birth. The second baby was asthmatic. The third baby had apparently normal health. The fourth baby was, like its mother, a problem child. On examination I found the following problems, listed below:

• Constant headaches.
• Dizzy spells.
• Blurred vision.
• Constant sore throat.
• Suspected thyroid dysfunction.
• 'Calcified' muscles.
• Pains across thorax.
• Right deltoid muscle enlarged, hard as if calcified and hot to the touch.
• Right arm mobility very restricted, lymphatic drainage restricted on thorax from the intercostals to the superficial muscles, dermis and epidermis.
• The abdominal cavity – nerve pain would not permit examination.
• Hips, lumbar region, sacrum, coccyx, trochanter, femur, knee joints, tibia and fibula, ankles and feet completely covered with what appeared to be a calcified mosaic pattern of vessels. The dermis down to the subcutaneous tissue on the heels cracked and had an offensive smell and bleeding.

The first few treatments were lengthy – three hours and more, with constant steam heat and very light treatment. By the end of each treatment she was exhausted (and so was I). I made sure I did not book any more patients after her on that day!

As treatment progressed on abdomen, two obstructions manifested. Medial to stomach and pancreas and the other at the transtubercular plane anterior to the aortic lymph glands. The two obstructions degenerated after a few treatments and did not come back.

She had been attended by her doctor for years and nothing more could be done to alleviate the condition, only to have the administration of drugs. A few months later the headaches ceased to worry her and the drug intake became unnecessary. Treatment would have to be demonstrated.

Sixteen months after her last treatment, she wrote me a note in which she stated: "Before I came to you I was taking eight painkillers a day just to get along. Since I came here, I haven't needed to take any. The pain I get now is only slight to what I used to have."

This person today leads a very active work and social life in her community, participating in charitable organisations, coaching the 8–10 year olds in tennis classes and playing lawn bowls. At the end of the season she received a gold medal from the association for being the outstanding player of the year in the league.

Multiple Sclerosis

I find I get good results from working on the deep lymphatics that are in close proximity to the deep nerve fibres and blood vessels. I have three copies of *Gray's Anatomy* – a revised edition (1904) of Henry Grays' 1901 book, the 35th edition, and the 37th edition. In the first edition, there is an illustration (fig. 342, p. 633) which shows how the deep lymphatics, vessels, nodes and plexuses surrounding the aortic artery appears similar to a 'lace pattern' covering the arteries and veins. The 35th and 37th editions do not have this illustration. The 35th edition has illustrations of lymphangiograms of the lymph vessels in the inguinals that have been injected with a dye. As the lymph vessels' drainage is blocked, as in the lymphangiogram, the nerve impulses from the brain to innervate all the muscle fibres in the body are fibrillated.

The nutrients, minerals, chemicals and water required by the body are transported to all parts by the oxygenated blood. The expansion and contraction of the blood vessels created by the cardiac cycle – systole, diastole and diastasis cordis – distributes the interstitial fluid, carried by the blood, into the interstitium, through the fenestrated muscles of the veins and capillaries. The above is repeated, on average, 72–80 times per minute. The denuded interstitial fluid, with the wastes of metabolism and foreign particulate, is pushed towards the deep valved, blind ending ducts of the lymphatics by the systolic pressure. It takes about five heartbeats to clear the debris through the valves, where it is fractionized, liquefied and neutralized. The blind ending ducts have the valves at the side of the vessels – these valves allow fluid to flow in only one direction to prevent a back flow. When the 'interstitial' fluid enters the lymph ducts, it is **then** termed **lymph fluid**.

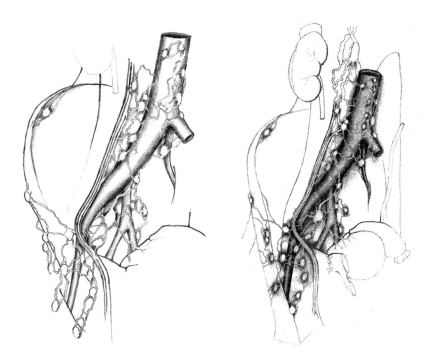

Figure 65: Two views of lymph drainage from perineum to kidneys.

If the interstitial fluid and blood flows have been slowed down by a blow, twist or injury, the fluid gels and the blood from the damaged veins and capillaries coagulates, because the rate of flow has been reduced from the normal rate of twenty feet per second. The pulsation of the blood is not strong enough to propel the interstitial fluid and nutrients through the normal channels and it bypasses the obstruction.

To my knowledge, both theory and practice, the injuries and subsequent results are the aetiological factor in most of the symptoms we observe in, for example, multiple sclerosis and varicosities.

When a tissue cell is ruptured, the nutrients, minerals and chemicals are mixed with the calcium contained in the interstitium. The phosphates stored in the mitochondria of the cell cause the fluids to calcify. This causes the white shadow to form that is seen in X-rays and scans and completely blocks the lymphatic flow traversing through the plexuses between the deep muscles on, and near, the bone, also at the top of the leg, inferior to the perineum. A weakness of the muscles prevails through nerve fibrillation.

To clear the musculature of the calcification, I work from the feet upwards, as the patient lies prone, in between the muscles both deep and superficial. If it does not overstress the patient, I follow the deep muscles and vessels at the origins and insertions of those deep muscles into the bone. Work both up and down, towards and away from the heart. It is a fallacy to work only towards the heart. Why is it there is always more oxygenated, nutrient-filled blood pulsated downwards than there is denuded venous blood, flowing back towards the heart? What is never taken into account is the way the cardiac cycle pulsates the nutrient-filled interstitial fluid from the bloodstream into the interstitium at systole, or in a downward direction. The multidirectional flow of interstitial fluid and lymphatic drainage required both directions of work to assist free drainage.

Practitioners should concentrate on the deep muscle fibres of the legs because of the degeneration caused by the calcification. I work on the feet first and then massage both ways to the knee. I then slightly curve the fingers of either hand, and pull downward from the perineum. This action helps to 'fracture' any calcified matter in the plexus at the superior part of the leg down to the adductor hiatus in the Hunter's canal. Then use flat-handed massage from the knee to the perineum. Repeat the above movements a few times, according to the chronicity of the complaint, and use hot foments. The plexus will then feel relaxed because the fractionized foreign particulate in the vessels will liquefy and flow into the perineum vessels to the glands. I then work flat-handed to massage the body to the cranium and we use the steam heat for the relaxation and liquefaction of the deep lymphatic debris. Some patients will react to an injury of a few months to a couple of years; others will not show any symptoms for up to thirty years. It is an advantage to have the treatment demonstrated and see how to use the hot foments to the best advantage.

Myositis Ossificans and Others

Below are the answers to many questions asked by practitioners in a training school in Melbourne, Victoria.

- "Are you familiar with myositis ossificans formation after a heavy blow to the periosteum? I ask this question because it is my understanding that any local treatment in the first few days only stimulates further osteoblastic activity, causing even greater depositions of bone."
- "What would you not treat?"

My assessment of the first question would be as follows. Immediately after an accident, the site of impact swells rapidly. If blood vessels and capillaries have been ruptured by the blow, the colour of the injury would be of venous blood permeating the tissues. If the dermis and epidermis have been damaged, some blood exudes, but mainly a plasma substance presents. A swelling on the periosteum is noted where the muscle fibres have been ruptured and pulled from the root canals in the bone. This assessment is made from what I feel as I work on the injury; blood will coagulate and the interstitial fluid will gel as the drainage is reduced to below twenty feet a second. The interstitial fluid consistency is half water and half plasma.

The injury on the cortical bone, subperiostal tissue and periosteum varies in size and shape, depending upon the object causing the injury, and there is always a hardened 'core' at the site. The tissues/muscles/tendons surrounding the core rapidly fill with fluid, i.e. tissue fluid, which consists of plasma, water and blood that has seeped from the broken vessels. It is well known that blood, interstitial fluid and lymph coagulate at the site of any injury.

If the blow was severe, depressions would be evident on the tuberosities and in the lacunae of the long bones. On the flat bones, a protuberance of a bone-like substance would form because of a leakage of bone protein through the injury and the presence of osteoblasts, a bone-forming cell.

When examining skeletons at the Medical School, I noted a large number of nutrient canals in all the bones, and in particular the long bones (the skeletal bones in the Medical School are not plastic). If the gelled fluid and coagulated blood remaining in the damaged bone and tissues is liquefied by the application of steam-heat and propelled into the deep blind-ended valved ducts by the cardiac cycle pulsation and specialized massage, the blood carrying nutrients for new bone growth and regeneration of the tissue cells, would again flow through the Volkmann's and Haversian canals. This would inhibit the inflammation and necrosis associated with this type of injury.

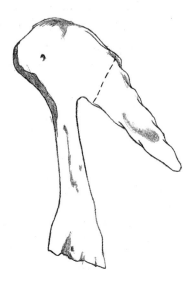

Figure 66: A bony spur at iliac crest of a quadriplegic patient.

With the liquefaction of the foreign particulate, it drains through between 8 and 10 lymph nodes to be purified by the 15 natural killer and filtration cells within the lymph node. Lymphocytes are produced in the bone marrow stem cells, lymph nodes and spleen. The lymphocytes, in conjunction with macrophages and phagocytes also function in surveillance and defense. Lymphocytes recognise foreign cells, microbes and other antibodies. The T cells destroy the foreign particulate by releasing various substances. The B cells differentiate into plasma cells and secrete antibodies that destroy the foreign particulate by fractionization, liquefaction and neutralization.

If, by the fibrillation of a nerve impulse caused by the accumulated debris from the blow, the strength of the impulse is decreased at the motor end plate, the irritability from the foreign particulate stimulates the muscle fibres with the acidic wastes from cellular metabolism, which reduces the strength of the contraction until it is too weak and is fatigued. I also find this phenomenon whilst treating arrhythmia and angina. These are described elsewhere. My thoughts on the above reaction would be similar to drug administration if the patient was allergic to the drug used.

As the strength of contraction becomes progressively less, the production of acetylcholene – a chemical that alters the muscle cell membrane as an electrical shock is diminished, as is the enzyme acetylcholinesterase that prevents the re-excitation of the muscle fibres until the next impulse – is lost as well.

The fibrillated muscle fibres retain the acetylcholine and acetylcholinesterase, which are not reabsorbed by the cellular tissues and causes a blockage. As a consequence of the muscle fibres failing to respond to the impulse, the foreign particulate remains within the fibres and lymphatic vessels where it calcifies. The calcium within the musculature at the fibrillation will enter the ruptured cells and mix with the phosphates stored in the mitochondria to form a calcification.

As a consequence of the muscles failing to respond to the weakened impulse, the calcification is noted in some form or other in all arthritic and rheumatic patients, including quadriplegia, which I have described elsewhere.

Again, by using the steam heated foments and specialized massage in the direction of the flow of body fluid drainage, the foreign particulate from the blow liquefies and drains through the appropriate channels.

In my many years of practising, I have encountered patients with old bruises. I find in the 'core' of the old bruise an obstruction of calcified matter. I query the length of time from presentation of injury to present. Some will only have the bruise a week or two whilst others will have had the discoloration for twenty-five years! It only takes one or two treatments to fractionize, liquefy and neutralize the debris. The colour is always a greenish-yellow and situated in the subcutaneous tissue.

Finally, my answer to the second question would be that I would not under any circumstances treat suspected appendix problems or a pregnancy.

Osteomyelitis

I treated a friend intermittently for about 18 months. He had 'everything and every problem' from head to toe. I noted the following problems:

1. Eyes, dull;
2. Sclera, red;
3. Drawn expression on face;
4. Red, blotchy, dry skin;
5. Glands in throat swollen and sore to touch, fluid retention;
6. Shoulders and arms sore;
7. Large swelling around root of neck;

8.   Large swelling on ribcage over diaphragm, which appeared to cause breathing problems;

9.   Pain in lymph plexuses lateral to umbilicus and extending through obliquus muscles to spine;

10. Lymph glands and vessels draining to and from inguinal nodes blocked as if calcified and hot to the touch;

11. Legs, plexus at top of leg blocked into perineum;

12. Large plaques of foreign particulate blocking interstitial fluid and lymph from draining back into nodes and glands in abdominal cavity;

13. Large painful varicosities in legs with calcified tissue surrounding the arteries and veins;

14. Large dark scars on legs from early lesions that had healed.

My first treatment was to sit the patient in a chair at the side of the plinth to rest the arms and shoulder muscles and relax the pressure on the origins and insertions of muscles and ligaments while I worked. I used steam heat and gentle flat-hand massage towards the transverse and spinous processes, apical and supraclavicular lymph plexuses at the root of the neck. I worked from the occipital bone downward between the spinous processes and the transverse spines, over and through the cervical muscles and ligaments of the cranial and cervical bones from the atlas, axis and lordotic curve to thoracic bones. I repeated the above procedure a few times with the steam heat pads. I then requested him to lie prone on the plinth for further treatment.

After a few treatments, chair first, then prone and supine on the plinth, lesions again manifested. I concentrated on treating the feet and legs to the perineum to

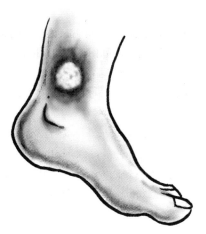

Figure 67: An osteomyelitis lesion.

penetrate the barrier of foreign particulate at the plexus in each leg, inferior to the perineum, which felt as if it had calcified. The secretion from the lesions was apparently the foreign particulate I had worked on in the plexus and it liquefied and 'overloadeded' the lymphatic vessels. The lesion was about 12mms in diameter and 10mms high. It differed in texture to an ordinary eruption, which is part liquid, cream coloured pus; it was a fatty, waxy, starchy translucent substance and came out in globules as if it was encased in a clear gelatinous coat, as an amyloid protein.

After the amyloid had been removed, an amber coloured plasma fluid drained from the lesion with a trace of blood for about 24 hours, when it healed, leaving a dark scar. Normally, blood will flow freely through the vascular system in the musculature, whereby nutrients are released through the fenestrated muscles of the veins and capillaries during the cardiac cycle. The fluid, which appears to be half water, half plasma, is called interstitial fluid and released into the interstitium to feed and bathe the tissue cells and bone. If the drainage is blocked, the healthy cells will necrotize. My questions have always been:

1.   What happens if this dysfunction occurs?
2.   What happens to the necrotized cells of bone and cellular tissue?

The only way I know to remove the degenerative cancer-forming particulate is to use steam heat and gentle flat-hand massage around any obstruction of the deep lymphatic vessels. I do not work through them as a whole by force to remove the necrotized cells, because the foreign particulate would only relocate to another vessel and form another growth with the potential to destroy the healthy cells surrounding the new obstruction.

By working on the blocked drainage, the interstitial fluid pulsated into the interstitium would gradually drain the foreign particulate during massage and the application of steam heat into the deep lymphatic vessels. Again, I used gentle massage with light probing if it was not too debilitating for the patient.

The shoulders, head and neck were treated first to clear the musculature and digestive glands and to help the lymphatic vessels to drain off the oedematous fluid. When this was achieved, I then concentrated on the feet and legs up to the perineum to heal the lesions. The fatty, waxy, starchy translucent amyloid protein, plus the excess water in the interstitium was drained from the lower limbs to allow the lesions to heal. The biggest problems encountered in the legs were the varicosities of the arteries and veins, and how to treat and avoid rupturing the blood vessels.

I overcame this successfully. Surrounding the veins, the cellular tissue had calcified or the amyloid protein had consolidated to the degree that every cardiac cycle expansion of the blood vessels would pulsate against either the calcification or degenerated amyloid protein and would lacerate the outer or epithelial coat of the vessels known as the tunica adventitia. The weakened walls in the veins, the tunica adventitia and the tunica media bulged to what could be described as a 'bunch of grapes' under the epidermis and dermis. The arteries were also weakened by the rupturing of the tunica adventitia, tunica media and tunica intima or endothelium.

I did a lot of massage on the legs and applied a lot of hot foments to liquefy the consolidated mass surrounding the blood vessels. The work and steam heat finally fractionized and liquefied the particulate to allow the vessel walls to regenerate to near normal size, eliminating any possibility of vessel rupture and seepage of blood into the interstitium.

The plexus surrounding the top of the leg, and from the superior aspect of the trochanter to the iliac crest which surround the inguinal nodes and glands anterior was calcified. I gave relief to this condition by using small heated pads from the sacrum, perineum and over the transtubercular plane. Both work and heat gave relief from the pain. The nodes and glands, deep and superficial, were both the size of a pea to a large broad bean. They had not drained normally for years. I associated the above with the use of bicycles – the hard and narrow seats would not be manufactured to specifications for large or tall, small or short stature. I have noted this problem with many patients who have leg and hip problems – some go back to childhood when they were trying to ride an adult-sized machine.

At this stage of healing, I released more toxic debris than the blocked drainage was capable of clearing through the plexuses. Lesions again formed on the ankles, gastrocnemius and the epicondyles of the femur. They discharged the amyloid protein, blood and water for about five and half days and then healed.

I had the root of the neck and surrounding lymphatics and the nodes and plexuses of the perineum almost free of exudate, so I started work on the abdominal cavity. As I worked over the intestines, liver, pancreas, spleen, duodenum, jejunum and diaphragm, the blood glucose level rose to 18.8. When this occurred, I again worked on the diaphragm and ribcage. After the first treatment, the blood glucose went down to 11.8 in July. Finally, in November, the glucose count was 4. It stabilised between 4 and 7 and has remained at that level since. The patient has kept twice-weekly records of sugar level since then. The treatment is described in more detail under the section on Diabetes Mellitus.

With the blood sugar level under control, the next problem manifested on the left patella. A friend of the patient had put hot foments on the blister that had formed and discharged some of the amyloid protein, blood and water. I worked exclusively on the leg for two hours, incorporating massage and steam heat from the inguinals to the knee, and foot to knee to discharge the foreign particulate through the lesion.

After about three applications of heat and work, the amyloid protein and other debris were drawn out. This left ten small lesions attached to the bone by what could have been either drainage vessels or small muscle attachments. The dead skin from the top of the blister degenerated and left the lesions exposed. Having cleaned and bandaged the wound, I then sent the patient home with instructions to come back the next day.

When I saw the patient again, the lesions had extruded the amyloid protein, but the outer tissue and its attachments to the bone remained. I again worked on the leg as I did the previous day and cleaned out the fluid exudate and put on another sterile dressing. Within the next twelve hours, the lesions and debris had disintegrated, leaving an open wound.

On the third day, after the initial work and heat, I again worked on the patella and noted the characteristic appearance of involcra (a coating or sheath) and sequestra from which blood and water seeped. The lesion on the bone was a V-shaped injury on the lateral side and deep. As I massaged and applied heat, the sequestrum (dead bone) separated from the healthy bone and flowed off like a grit or sand, into the deep lymphatic drainage.

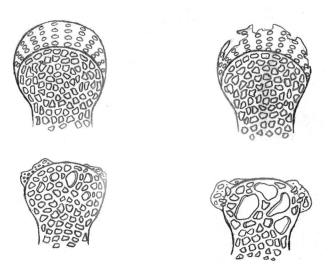

Figure 68: An osteoporotic degradation caused by amyloid protein blocking canals in bone preventing the absorption of nutrition.

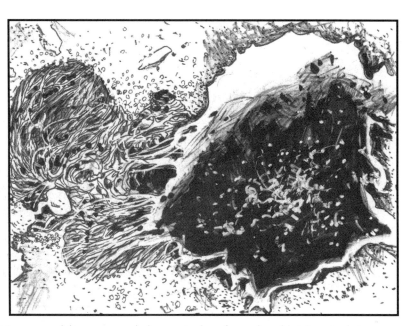

Figure 69: The resorption of cortical bone caused by blocked canals preventing the absorption of nutrients. The bone resorbs cortical bone from one area to cover another exposed area, leaving the collagen fibres without support.

Massage and heat removed the particulate from the old injury and the wound healed within four days. Very little scarring remains. After the debris was cleared from the triangular injury, I noted a depression on the patella that extended through the anterior cortical bone and trabeculated bone, leaving only a thin cortical layer on its posterior surface.

All medical evidence shows it was classical haematogenous osteomyelitis with the degradation of bone. With treatment, it only took a few days to repair and renew the damaged area.

Osteoporosis

I have had many patients who have suffered from this debilitating disease. I noted in the initial treatments one prevailing factor – the vertebrae are the most affected part of the skeleton. If left untreated, the whole system degenerates.

It first appears to be caused by the fibrillation of the central nervous system and peripheral nerves from the dysfunction of the deep lymphatic vessels. As I work on the body, I note there is an amyloid – a starchy, fatty, waxy, translucent protein which is produced in the brain and deposited in tissues as it drains out of the arachnoid space of the medulla. This blocks the interstitial fluid from entering the nutrient canals of bone. Amyloid protein is insoluble and is impervious to lymphatic purification.

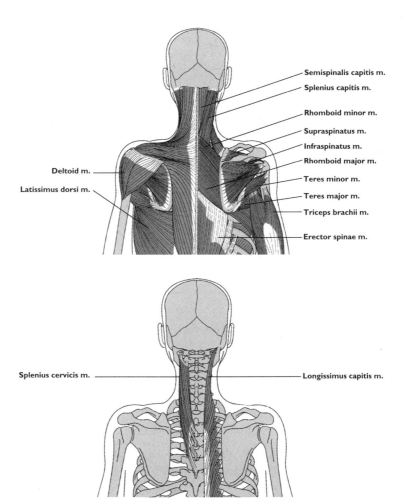

Semispinalis capitis m.

Splenius capitis m.

Rhomboid minor m.

Supraspinatus m.

Infraspinatus m.

Rhomboid major m.

Teres minor m.

Teres major m.

Triceps brachii m.

Erector spinae m.

Deltoid m.

Latissimus dorsi m.

Splenius cervicis m.

Longissimus capitis m.

Figure 70: The nerves at the base of the skull fibrillate through blocked drainage causing calcification.

The bone, through the lack of nutrition from the interstitial fluid, will react by reabsorbing protein from existing bone from one part and laying it down in another section. This is the conclusion I arrived at when I massaged the affected area; some parts are smooth as if normal and others have a recess or depression on the surface.

I treat the condition the same as I do arthritis because, although the amyloid protein resists the fractionization, liquefaction and neutralization of the lymphatic system, it will liquefy as I apply the steam-heated pads, and flow off in the direction of the drainage as I massage the affected parts.

It is a slow process, but it eventually clears once the nutrient canals can again transport the nutrients to the affected bone. One of my patients, now in her seventies, was down to 56 bone density when I started her treatment; when I finished, it was up to 88.5. She is still alive and happy at the time of writing and I still hear from her occasionally. The protein marker in urine represents the amount of bone shed and not replaced.

Parkinson's Disease

Parkinson's disease (also known as paralysis agitans) is named after the London general practitioner, James Parkinson, who described the condition in 1817. I note the first sign of the above condition is a stiffening of muscles causing a fibrillation of the cranial nerves controlling the head, neck, shoulders and arms, inhibiting control of movement.

As the 'disease' advances, the tremors increase and involve the musculature of the body. The head and back leans forward with little or no control. The first system I examine is the deep lymphatic pathways from the head to the feet. My questions are:

1.   What causes the dysfunction?
2.   What causes the calcification at the base of the skull?
3.   What causes the fibrillation of the cranial nerves as they pass through the foramina at the base of the skull lateral to foramen magnum?
4.   What causes the calcified obstructions surrounding the semispinalis capitis insertion at the occipital bone, splenius capitis insertion into temporal bone and longissimus capitis also inserted into the temporal bone?

I have found that this problem is caused by an accident or a severe head movement which results in whiplash. The fine roots of the muscles and the transverse ligament of the atlas and axis are either torn out of the root canals of bone or ruptured. Bone protein will leak from the injury; the dead bone cells which form a powdery sand will mix with the calcium in the tissue fluid and penetrate the ruptured tissue cells. It will then combine with the phosphates stored in the mitochondria of those cells to form a calcification. The obstructions arising from the calcification are classified as 'loose bodies', the irregular shaped 'bone' as seen in X-rays. I treat Parkinson's disease as I would Hodgkin's disease as they both involve the dysfunction of the deep lymphatic vessels surrounding the cranial, cervical, thoracic and peripheral nerves. Treatment would have to be demonstrated for an effective cure.

Stomach Complaints

The wall of the stomach and intestines is covered in a thick layer of mucus to withstand the action of the acids as they break down the nutrients, chemicals and minerals ingested. About one and a half litres of acids and digestive juices are produced every twenty-four hours for an average size individual.

No diet will prevent stomach complaints. A 'bloated' or 'nauseous' condition is caused by a dysfunctioning digestive system. To find the basic cause, I examine the glands in the cheeks, throat and mouth, which produce the digestive juices. The main elements are:

• The mouth. Secretes saliva, which reduces food to a fluid and supplies mucus or serous fluid and ptyaline (alpha amylase).
• Parotid glands. Produces saliva or serous fluid.
• Submaxillary. Saliva.
• Sublingual. Saliva.
• Labial and buccal glands. In cheeks; glands of mixed types.
• Lingual glands in tongue. Mucus.
• Palatine glands in roof of mouth. Mucus.
• Oesophagus. Mucus.
• Fundus glands – gastric. Contains mucus, zymogenic cells which produce pepsinogen and parietal cells.

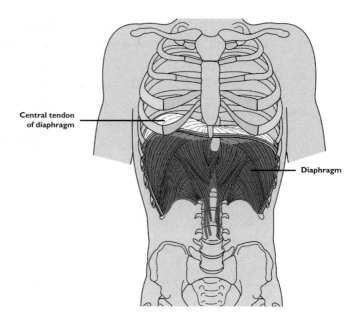

Central tendon
of diaphragm

Diaphragm

Figure 71: The diaphragm creates peristalsis by inspiration / expiration of air in the lungs. This action is also required to innervate the oesophagus and intestines.

- Pepsinogen. A zymogen – a precursor of pepsin – a protein digesting enzyme. Also converted into active enzyme by the action of an acid, pepsin, a proteolytic enzyme, which is a digestive component of gastric juice. It is formed from pepsinogen by acids.
- Hydrochloric acid (HCl). One of the substances contained in gastric juice; also sulphate – an ester of sulphuric acid. HCl in stomach.
- Stomach glands. Cardiac and pyloric glands – occurring in cardiac and pyloric portions of stomach.
- Duodenum. Own glands and contributions from liver and pancreas (alkaline).
- Villi. Mucus secreting cells – contains a lacteal – a fine extension of the lymphatic system. Absorbs the sugars and amino acids. Lacteals accept fatty acids.
- Carbohydrates. Starches, lactose and sucrose – acted upon by (alpha amylase).
- Pancreatic amylase. An intestinal amylase in the small intestine.
- Monosaccharides, (glucose, galactose, fructose), absorbed from small intestinal walls into the bloodstream.
- Fats. Emulsified by bile salts, bile pigments and alpha amylase by agitation within the liver.
- Pancreatic enteric lipase. A fat splitting enzyme that forms glycerol and fatty acids.
- Bile. A mixture of bile salts and pigments.
- Pancreas. See full description in diabetes mellitus.

The glands retain a 'build-up' of acids and foreign particulate through the blocked drainage in the dysfunctioning deep lymphatic vessels. The peristaltic action of the oesophagus and diaphragm is absent and the 'build-up' of the foreign particulate inhibits the nerve innervation from the brain to the musculature; basically causing problems in the liver, pancreas, spleen, kidneys and intestines.

Peristaltic Action of the Oesophagus, Intestines and Diaphragm

A gastric ulcer occurs when the acid in the gastric juice corrodes the mucous membrane of the stomach and intestines because of little or no peristaltic action in the oesophagus, intestines and diaphragm.

The inhibited peristaltic action of the diaphragm occurs when the deep lymphatic vessels, nodes and plexuses drainage blocks on the ribcage in the upward flow of fluid to the subclavian veins via the inframammary plexus under the breast.

The 'build-up' of acids and foreign particulate block the deep blind ending valved ducts of the lymphatics particularly through the plexuses and vessels at the root of the neck and mediastinum in the thorax. The cranial nerves and the left and right phrenic nerve, a major branch of the cervical plexus, are attached to the cervicals down to the roots of the neck. The phrenic nerve then innervates the root of the lungs, passes through the bottom lobes of both lungs and attaches to each side of the diaphragm. It is the main nerve of inspiration/respiration of the lungs and the peristaltic action of the diaphragm and oesophagus. The rhythmic pulsation pushes the diaphragm down onto the abdominal viscera and organs and up onto the lobes of the lungs to expire the fluid and gases accumulated in the pulmonary alveoli.

The musculature in the centre of the diaphragm resembles a cloverleaf and is surrounded by muscle fibres that attach to the ribs, spine and sternum. It is a musculo-membranous partition separating the thoracic and abdominal cavities.

The inhibited peristaltic action of the diaphragm occurs when the deep lymphatic vessels, nodes and plexuses drainage blocks on the ribcage in the upward flow when the normal flow of fluid is slowed down below twenty ft/second. The plasma content in the interstitial and lymphatic fluid gels and prevents the diaphragm muscles from clearing the foreign particulate from the striations of muscle fibres.

The interstitial fluid within the striations of muscles flows back through the crural muscles to the thoracic duct. The interstitial fluid within the outer muscles that are attached to the ribs, sternum and spine drains out and upwards over the ribcage, into the deep lymphatic vessels that flow into the subclavian veins.

Peristalsis is initiated by the inspiration and expiration of air. At inspiration, the diaphragm muscles are extended and pushed onto the stomach, digestive organs and intestines as the air expands in the lungs. The pressure of this expansion helps to move the mixture of digested and half-digested food with the acids, alkalis and other digestive juices over the villi in the intestinal walls by rhythmic pulsation. It is then deposited into the mesenteric lymphatics at the side of the intestines by the villi and transported by the blood in the portal vein through the porta hepatis into the liver. The lipids are then processed back to water by agitation of bile salts, bile pigments and alpha amylase. It is then drained from the liver by the hepatic vein into the heart for distribution to the cells and bone by the interstitial fluid.

When the expiration occurs, the respiratory muscles relax and allow the diaphragm to return the chest cavity to its minimum size to expel gases and fluids collected in the lungs from inspiration.

When the peristaltic action of the diaphragm is inhibited through deep lymphatic blockage, the nerve impulse activating the musculo-membranous fibres is fibrillated. The result of this retains the excess fluids and foreign particulate within the striations of muscles. When this problem occurs, the normal action of the diaphragm is lost and the gas inhibiting cells in the intestinal walls do not function.

The acids and partially digested food remain in the stomach and intestines, which causes ulcers to form. The gaseous content and fluid retained in the lungs will affect breathing, which affects the inspiration of oxygen to maintain normal functions of the brain, heart, lungs and body organs.

With the occurrence of a gastric ulcer and other debilitating problems, it is of no advantage to drink milk to effect a cure – it will only give temporary relief. It is also a misconception that a gastric ulcer is caused by stress. Tension will induce the production of acids from the foreign particulate and partially digested food, but is not the cause of the complaint. I find the precursor to be the body wastes/toxins blocked in the dysfunctioning **deep** lymphatics surrounding the digestive glands and the diaphragm.

Some common culprits being ingested are highly spiced foods, fatty foods, and other gas-forming products, such as onions, garlic, leeks, peas, cabbage, cauliflower, broccoli and some acidic fruits as well as some nuts. Acidic tomatoes, cucumbers and lettuce will also, at times, create the same problems. Patients suffering from any stomach complaint caused by the above will not find any relief or long-term cure from gastric or any other pain by ingesting drugs or any specialized diet.

Treatment

When the digestive system dysfunctions, the first place I look at and treat is the glands from the occipital to the root of the neck. If a patient has had any injury to the head and neck, the lymphatic drainage will gel if the flow has been slower than 20 feet per second. Interstitial fluid flow is also affected. The gel and debris from cellular tissue and bone protein will decompose and will emit a taste and smell like detritus from decayed teeth. The foreign particulate being held in and around the digestive glands at body temperature will prevent normal digestion. This then, with the excess of acids, forms a gas, which will cause a bloating and/or dysfunction causing the stomach and intestines to inflate. The pressure of the gas stretches the mucous lining of the viscera, creating a weakness for the acids and other foreign particulate to penetrate and cause ulcers and other growths to form.

To treat, I sit the patient in a chair, preferably at the side of the plinth to relax their shoulder and arm muscles. I initiate work from the occipital to the root of the neck; apply one or two sets of hot foments between the massage. The deep lymphatic vessels, nodes and plexuses should be relaxed sufficiently to allow the gelled fluid to drain from the affected areas. I then request the patient to lie prone on the plinth. I work from the feet upwards, through the legs to the perineum with the same procedure, using light work and steam heat from the pads to relax the deep lymphatic vessels and gelled fluid to flow in through the perineum.

I find when I release the blocked drainage at the root of the neck and the perineum, the flow of both interstitial and lymph fluid will disperse because then, if the ulcer breaks before it is ready, there is the possibility another ulcer will form in the damaged area. Use the steam heat from the hot foments to liquefy and drain the pustular secretion into the apex of the lesion where it will implode. I treat this daily until the patient gets relief, which may only be two or three days. **Do not work through an ulcer; gently work around it.**

The first reaction a patient will have is an irritating itch in the throat, at or above the root of the neck. As they cough to relieve the irritation, this may well lead to vomiting – the foreign particulate vomited will be about two tablespoons of black coagulated blood with a yellow pustular secretion mixed in it. When this is released, a trace of oxygenated blood will follow and it will then stop. The second day, the irritation again manifests, but only about a teaspoon of coagulated blood will be released. Again, just a show of oxygenated blood. By the third day, there will be the same irritation but only a few spots of black blood; nothing else.

I usually request a patient to observe the colour of the faecal matter, and whether it is like a black sludge, for about 3 days; not every patient reacts by vomiting. After vomitus and faecal matter is released, the deep lymphatics will then fractionize, liquefy and neutralize any wastes, and the ulcer heals and does not recur.

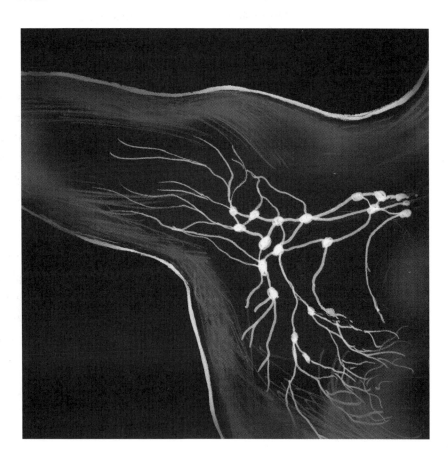

Figure 72: The lymph plexus shows the upward flow of fluid within the nodes and vessels.

Interstitial fluid drains into the lymphatics and it is propelled into the deep lymphatic glands within the abdominal cavity and thorax that fractionizes, liquefies and neutralizes the foreign particulate within the fluid. The nerve fibres that have been fibrillated by the blocked drainage as above will again innervate the motor end plates in the musculature. **To treat, work around the ulcer.**

To my knowledge, there are fifteen natural killer and agranular cells in a lymph node. They are:

Fibroblasts	Collagenoblasts
Plasma cells	Heterophils
Chondroblasts	Phagocytes
Granulocytes	Basophils
Trabeculae	Primitive reticular cells
Neutrophils	Macrophages
Lymphocytes (small)	Reticulocytes
Oesinophils	

There could be more as there are also lymphocytes (medial) and lymphocytes (large) that are NK cells. At first, I did not understand, or believe, there were as many cells within a node, but when I saw an enlarged specimen cut in its transverse diameter in solution at medical school anatomy section, I had to revise my thoughts. I would like to have seen it cut longitudinally. The lymph fluid and foreign particulate passes through between 8 and 10 lymph nodes to be fractionized, liquefied and neutralized before it re-enters the bloodstream.

The deep cervical group of lymph nodes is formed by the union of the various chains of lymph nodes. There are also numerous lymph nodes scattered along the jugular vein with a meshwork of vessels. The meningeal lymphatics of the brain pass through the foramen in the occipital with the cranial nerve fibres and empty into the deep cervical chains. The cerebral lymphatics drain through the foramen magnum and they too empty into the deep cervical chains.

To treat the deep cervical group, the practitioner must wear surgical gloves as the cricoid/thyroid bone is pushed sideways to locate the groove between the spine and the bones. The fingers should be gently inserted into the groove and worked downwards to relieve the pressure of the blocked drainage of the cranial nerve fibres that cause the fibrillation. Steam heat is essential for this particular treatment as it liquefies the foreign particulate that fibrillates the nerves which innervate the eyes, ears, nose, throat, heart, lungs, diaphragm and viscera. Treatment must be demonstrated to those who would wish to practise this.

Some patients whose sight has deteriorated will have bright flashes of light, which will fluctuate, and have a taste and smell in their mouth and nose, like detritis from decayed teeth. There is also an expectoration of colloidin which will be an amber/brown colour with streaks of green and yellow mucus that has an offensive smell.

Other patients suffering from migraine headaches accompanied by a nauseous reaction will have an ectopic calcification at the occipital/atlas facets that mainly arise from some injury; for example, a car accident. Care has to be taken because of the fibrillation of the cranial nerves. Initially, I do gentle massage with the steam heat, as I would treat arthritis.

If the alpha amylase (ptyaline), secreted in the saliva by HCl (hydrochloric acid), the pancreatic amylase and intestinal amylase are absent in the mesenteric lipids, there is nothing to assist the bile salts and pigments to agitate the lipids to water for its return to the bloodstream. The lipids are then transported to the heart via the hepatic vein. As the blood is pulsated through the vascular system by the cardiac cycle systole, diastole and diastasis cordis, the interstitial fluid is filtered out through the fenestrated muscles of the veins and capillaries into the interstitium. The ingested lipids that have been filtered out of the interstitial fluid remain within the walls of the blood vessels and cause a cholesterol build--up, slowing down or blocking the blood flow. I observed this in specimens in solution at the medical school.

The liver, with the excess of lipids, will show in X-rays and scans to be enlarged. The patient will vomit which will be a green slime and full of lipids.
An acidic fatty taste is noted by patient and the nauseous feeling will still prevail.

To treat the 'upset stomach', as previously quoted, the patient sits in a chair by the plinth first, then lies prone on plinth and work is initiated from feet to head, with the use of steam heat. The patient then lies supine and treatment is repeated from the feet to the head, using the steam heat, following the direction of the lymphatic drainage from the liver and diaphragm. The steam heat liquefies the lipids and the massage will drain the particulate into the bloodstream where it is then pulsated into the kidneys and voided at micturition.

Bibliography

Anderson, P.D.: Clinical Anatomy and Physiology for Allied Health Sciences.

Bergland, R.: 1985. Fabric of Mind.

Clemente, C.D.: 1987. Anatomy 3rd Edition.

Crocco, J.A: 1977. Gray's Anatomy – Classic Collector's Edition, First printed in 1901.

da Vinci, L: Primer on the Rheumatic Diseases, 8th Edition. From the Royal Library, Windsor Castle.

DeCoursey, R.M.: 1961. The Human Organism, 2nd Edition.

Gray, H.: 1973. Gray's Anatomy, 35th Edition.

Gray, H.: 1975. Gray's Anatomy, 37th Edition.

Atlas of the Body and Mind, Mitchell Beazley, 1976.

Illustrated World of Science Encyclopaedia, books 1–3, 1971.

McClintic, J.R: 1983. Human Anatomy, 1st Edition.

McMinn, R.M.H., Hutchings, R.T., Logan, B.M.: 1981. Head and Neck Anatomy.

Miller, B.F., Kean, C.B.: 1983. Encyclopedia and Dictionary of Medicine, Nursing and Allied Health Sciences.

Revell, P.A.: 1986. Pathology of Bone.

Ross & Wilson: 1973. Foundations of Anatomy and Physiology, 4th Edition.

Rowett, H.G.Q.: Basic Anatomy and Physiology, 2nd Edition.

Thibodeau, G.A., Patton, G. A.: 1999. Anatomy and Physiology, 4th Edition.

Tortora, G. J., Anagnostakos, N. P.: 1990. Principles of Anatomy and Physiology, 6th Edition

Weston, T.: 1988. Atlas of Anatomy.

Yoffrey, J. M., Courtice F.C.: 1970. Lymphatics, Lymph and the Lymphomyeloid Complex.

Notes